THE BIOLOGY OF AIDS
Fourth Edition

W9-CHA-845

Hung Fan
Ross F. Conner
Luis P. Villarreal

University of California, Irvine

JONES AND BARTLETT PUBLISHERS
Sudbury, Massachusetts
BOSTON   TORONTO   LONDON   SINGAPORE

World Headquarters
Jones and Bartlett Publishers
40 Tall Pine Drive
Sudbury, MA 01776
978-443-5000
info@jbpub.com
www.jbpub.com

Jones and Bartlett Publishers Canada
2100 Bloor Street West
Suite 6-272
Toronto, ON M6S 5A5
Canada

Jones and Bartlett Publishers International
Barb House, Barb Mews
London, W6 7PA
UK

Library of Congress Cataloging-in-Publication Data
Fan, Hung, 1947–
    The Biology of AIDS/Hung F. Fan, Ross F. Conner, and Luis P. Villarreal.—4th ed.
        p.   cm.
    Includes index.
    ISBN 0-7637-1116-0 (pbk.)
    1. AIDS (Disease)   I. Conner, Ross F.   II. Villarreal, Luis P.
III. Title.
RC607.A26.F35   2000
616.97'92—dc21

                                                                99-059503

VP, College Editorial Director: Brian L. McKean
Production Editor: Linda DeBruyn
Product Marketing Manager: Elizabeth Pearson
Editorial/Production Assistant: Anne Trafton
Director of Production and Design: Anne Spencer
Director of Manufacturing: Therese Bräuer
Cover Design: Stephanie Torta
Typesetting: Nesbitt Graphics, Inc.
Printing and Binding: Malloy Lithography

Cover Photo Credit: Copyright © 1999 Photodisc

Printed in the United States of America

03   02   01   00   10   9   8   7   6   5   4   3   2   1

To our HIV-infected friends and acquaintances who are courageously battling the disease or who have succumbed to it. In their honor, and to hasten the day when this book is no longer necessary, a portion of the royalties from this book will be donated to foundations and community organizations dedicated to AIDS research and service.

BRIEF CONTENTS

CONTENTS

CHAPTER 5

Clinical Manifestations of AIDS 79

PREFACE

The purpose of this text is to provide the nonspecialized student with a firm overview of AIDS from a biomedical perspective. The biological aspects include cellular and molecular descriptions of the immune system and the AIDS virus (human immunodeficiency virus, or HIV). The consequences of HIV infection from cell to organism are also covered, along with a clinical description of the disease. These topics can be covered only in a survey fashion due to the comprehensive nature of this approach and the additional aim of making this text appropriate for a one-quarter (or semester) course (or part of such a course). We focus first on presenting the relevant fundamental principles. Following a brief presentation of these principles for each topic, we generalize and apply these concepts to the case of AIDS.

The Biology of AIDS was first published in 1989. Two subsequent, updated editions followed. We then expanded the book to include psychosocial aspects of HIV/AIDS, and it was published as *AIDS: Science and Society* (first and second editions). During the planning stage for the third edition of *AIDS: Science and Society*, we decided to reintroduce *The Biology of AIDS* to meet the needs of those more specifically focused on AIDS from a biomedical perspective. *The Biology of AIDS, Fourth Edition* represents the biomedical chapters of *AIDS: Science and Society, Third Edition*. We have updated and written new sections in several chapters and provided the latest available statistics on AIDS as the book went to press. We have also added a reference appendix in which students can obtain additional information on AIDS. A major feature of this appendix is the inclusion of several Web sites students can explore to find up-to-date information about AIDS. Jones and Bartlett has also established a Web site that is linked to this book (www.jbpub.com/AIDS). This Web site will be updated periodically with new developments in both the biomedical and social aspects of AIDS.

This book is patterned after a one-quarter course, AIDS Fundamentals, taught at the University of California, Irvine. Approximately half the course covers biomedical aspects of AIDS, and the other half covers social issues raised by the disease. The text represents the material covered in the first half of the course. At UCI, AIDS Fundamentals is open to all undergraduate students and is taught with the assumption that they have had a high school level modern-biology course. The material contained in Chapters 3 (immunology), 4 (virology), and 6 (epidemiology) is covered in three hours of lecture per chapter. Material covered in the other chapters is taught in a single one and one-half hour lecture per chapter. We have found that students are able to assimilate and retain the material when delivered at this rate. The course includes another important component: small discussion groups led by students who previously took the class. These peer-led groups use experiential exercises as a catalyst for a deeper understanding of the human and social aspects of HIV and AIDS. Another important feature of the AIDS Fundamentals course is two panel presentations by people affected by HIV/AIDS: a panel of people living with AIDS and a panel of HIV/AIDS health care workers.

Most researchers and scholars in AIDS-related fields were unprepared for the dramatic impact of the AIDS epidemic when it emerged in 1981. As virologists and social scientists, we might have expected modern biomedical technology to provide a quick technical solution or to at least prevent, through vaccine development, the spread of this major new viral epidemic. It is now clear that even though this technology has hastened biomedical progress in AIDS, the AIDS epidemic poses new and unforeseen difficulties with no quick biological solution in sight. These difficulties challenge both our scientific abilities and the ability of our society to respond appropriately. It is our goal to provide students with a conceptual framework of the issues raised by the AIDS epidemic so that they will be better able to deal with the challenges posed by this disease. This is particularly important because new information about scientific aspects of AIDS appears almost daily; with this information come new implications for the clinical, social, psychological, legal, and ethical aspects of the disease. We hope that the framework provided in this book will help students understand and make informed decisions about AIDS-related issues as they develop in the future.

ACKNOWLEDGMENTS

We wish to thank David Fan, Elaine Vaughan, Michael Gorman, David Prescott, Cedric Davern, David Baltimore, and Frank Lilly for reading parts of the original manuscript and providing many helpful substantive and editorial comments. Kathryn Radke and Ian Trowbridge provided helpful suggestions for a past revision; Ian also provided the content for the website linked to this book.

Special thanks to the following reviewers who provided comments on the last edition and advice for this revision:

Robert Fullilove, Columbia University

James D. Haynes, State University College at Buffalo

James Rothenberger, University of Minnesota

Ian Trowbridge, Salk Institute

Thomas C. Van Cott, Henry M. Jackson Foundation

Juan Moreno applied outstanding computer graphic skills in generating all the line drawings for the book. Bob Settineri of Sierra Productions was of great help in obtaining the other figures. Brian McKean, Anne Trafton, Linda DeBruyn, and other editorial staff of Jones and Bartlett were responsible for production of the final volume. We are grateful for their assistance and gentle prodding. We also wish to thank Michael Feldman and Emmett Carlson for their love and support.

AUTHORS

Dr. Hung Fan is Professor of Virology in the Department of Molecular Biology and Biochemistry at the University of California, Irvine and Director of the UCI Cancer Research Institute. His research interest is in how retroviruses cause disease and induce cancer and AIDS.

Dr. Ross Conner is Associate Professor, Department of Urban and Regional Planning, School of Social Ecology, and Department of Medicine, School of Medicine at the University of California, Irvine. Dr. Conner's research interest is in the evaluation of the effectiveness of public and social programs, particularly health promotion programs, including HIV prevention.

Dr. Luis Villarreal is Professor of Virology in the Department of Molecular Biology and Biochemistry at the University of California, Irvine. Dr. Villarreal's research interest is in the strategy of how viruses replicate and how they cause disease.

CHAPTER 1

Introduction:
An Overview of AIDS

A report appeared in 1981 that initially drew little attention from infectious disease experts. In that report, Dr. Michael Gottlieb, at the University of California at Los Angeles, described a rare form of pneumonia occurring in homosexual men. Other reports from about the same time indicated that other homosexual men were developing rare forms of cancer. This new set of symptoms, a *syndrome* in medical terms, was eventually called *acquired immune deficiency syndrome* because the symptoms were consistent with damage to the immune system in previously healthy individuals. Moreover, this disease was not congenital or inherited but appeared to have been acquired. We now know that this resulted from infection by a virus. Since then, the acronym *AIDS,* which is used to describe this disease, has become a prominent and permanent fixture in our language. It evokes a range of responses, including fear, hate, and mistrust. Some of these responses (hate, mistrust) are related to the association of AIDS with subcultural groups within our society, such as male homosexuals, who already have experienced discrimination. Other responses (fear) are due to the grave nature of the AIDS disease and the threat it may pose to society. This is because the AIDS epidemic continues to grow—unlike most other major infectious diseases, which have been controlled by a combination of clinical treatments and public health measures.

AIDS IN BRIEF

We now know that AIDS is caused by *human immunodeficiency virus (HIV),* but it was originally observed by its effects on the immune system. An important clue was that AIDS patients often developed a lung infection (or pneumonia) caused by a fungus called *Pneumocystis carinii.* This infection is very rare in healthy individuals, but patients with cancers of the immune system (lymphomas) were known to be susceptible to this disease. Lymphomas are usually treated by chemotherapy, which is intended to destroy the cancer cells. However, chemotherapy also unavoidably destroys many healthy immune cells along with the cancerous lymphoma cells. Thus, this type of pneumonia predominantly occurs in patients with damaged immune systems. Examination of AIDS patients confirmed that their immune systems were damaged. The specific nature of this damage is discussed in greater detail in Chapters 3 and 4. It had been known for some time that various other viral infections could damage cells of the immune system, but the severe damage seen with AIDS was unprecedented. Although doctors suspected early on that AIDS resulted from infection by a virus, it was not until 1984 that the virus was finally isolated by both French and American researchers. That virus is now known as *HIV*.

In addition to pneumonia, AIDS is associated with numerous other infections. These secondary infections are caused by various bacteria, protozoa, fungi, and other viruses. Usually, it is these infections (known as *opportunistic infections*) that cause death in AIDS patients. In addition to secondary infections, AIDS patients frequently develop cancers, including *lymphomas* and an otherwise rare cancer called *Kaposi's sarcoma*. HIV infection also can result in damage to brain cells. This leads to loss of mental function, referred to as *AIDS dementia*. A more complete description of the clinical features of AIDS is presented in Chapter 5. Most of these opportunistic infections and some other effects of HIV infection can be explained by damage to the immune system.

HIV causes disease insidiously. The early stages of infection may not be noticed by the infected individual. The infected person may feel healthy and appear to be completely normal during this time (the asymptomatic period), but such a person is able to transmit the infection. The HIV *incubation period* (the time between initial infection and appearance of disease) is of variable duration and can be quite long (on average, 10 years or more). In contrast, for most common viral infections, such as colds or influenza, an incubation period of a few days or weeks is followed by apparent disease. This adds greatly to the difficulty of studying and controlling AIDS, because many people infected with the virus have not yet developed the disease.

THE AIDS EPIDEMIC

Despite the many different clinical symptoms that result from AIDS, medical investigators know a great deal about how AIDS is spread in our population. For example, it is now clear that HIV transmission requires close contact and that infection occurs by one of three routes: blood, birth, or sex. Casual contact does not lead to disease transmission. These issues are further discussed in Chapter 7.

Between 1981 (the beginning of the AIDS epidemic) and 1997, about 641,000 cases of AIDS in the United States were reported to the national Centers for Disease Control and Prevention (CDCP) in Atlanta, Georgia. Of these cases, about 385,000 (60 percent) have died. Sexually active homosexual males were originally the major afflicted group and currently represent about 48 percent of these reported cases. Another 26 percent of the cases were male or female injection drug users, and 6 percent were male homosexual drug users. Another 14 percent resulted from heterosexual transmission, birth, or by blood transfusion during the period when the American blood supply was not monitored for HIV antibodies (1981–1985).

In the relatively brief period since the beginning of the AIDS epidemic, AIDS has already had a major impact on death and disease in the United States. Currently, there are between 40,000 and 60,000 new cases of HIV infection every year, and the number of people dying from AIDS per year is currently approximately 20,000. In comparison, approximately 40,000 women die each year from breast cancer, and about 35,000 men die each year from prostate cancer. On the other hand, the average age of death from breast or prostate cancer is considerably older than for death from AIDS. The AIDS epidemic has had a particularly high impact on African Americans and Hispanics, who show rates of HIV infection that are three to six times higher than that of the general population.

The AIDS epidemic is not restricted to the United States. It can be found on all continents and hence is considered a *pandemic*. It is estimated that 24 million people in sub-Saharan Africa are infected with HIV. In Africa, HIV transmission predominantly results from heterosexual contact and other modes. Given the relatively poor medical support available in much of Africa, the number of infected people may increase significantly. Recently, HIV infection has been spreading explosively in South Asia as well, with Thailand and India strongly affected. As there is no cure for AIDS, these numbers are alarming. They indicate the clear potential of AIDS to spread unchecked, despite recent advances in modern medicine, epidemiology, virology, and recombinant DNA technology. This reminds us of earlier times when major infectious diseases devastated human populations (see Chapter 2).

Worldwide, AIDS now ranks as the fourth leading cause of death after heart disease, strokes, and acute lower respiratory infections. In Africa, it is the leading cause of death. How can we control this epidemic? An overview of the relationship between epidemics and human populations may shed some light on this concern.

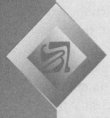

CHAPTER 2

Concepts of Infectious Disease and a History of Epidemics

One of the great recent achievements of modern civilization has been the control of infectious diseases. It is unlikely that many of us personally knew someone who died from a contagious disease. In historical terms, this is a new development, one that occurred in the twentieth century. In previous centuries, death from infectious disease was common, and whole populations were often affected.

When a population becomes infected with a contagious disease, an epidemic results. *Epidemic* derives from Greek and means "in one place among the people." To understand how an infectious disease can spread or remain established in a population, we must consider the relationship between an infectious disease agent and its host population. The study of diseases in populations is an area of medicine known as *epidemiology,* and is further discussed in Chapter 6.

We now know that contagious diseases are spread by microorganisms, such as certain bacteria and viruses, that cause disease when they infect a susceptible person. This is a modern concept, known as the *germ theory* of infectious disease. As we shall see, earlier societies often used moral or religious explanations for infectious disease, and their social behavior reflected those beliefs.

FACTORS THAT AFFECT THE SPREAD OF EPIDEMICS

In this section, we discuss factors that influence the spread of infectious diseases. Although various microorganisms cause disease, and the general principles are the same, we will concentrate on viruses, since HIV is a virus.

Host and Virus Populations

An epidemic consists of infection of a number of individuals in a population. It is important to look at more than a single person to understand how diseases spread. Two populations must be considered: the human host and the infecting agent—in the case of AIDS, a virus. These two populations have a balanced parasite–host relationship. A viral infection can deplete or limit the population of its host, but a highly lethal virus that spreads rapidly might kill all available hosts and lead to the extinction of both its host and itself. The outcome of an epidemic, however, is not always straightforward and can vary according to a number of other factors that relate to the population. These factors include:

1. the total number of hosts
2. their birth rate
3. the rate at which susceptible individuals migrate into the population
4. the number of susceptible hosts who are not infected
5. the rate at which the disease can be transmitted from an infected individual to an uninfected one
6. the number of infected individuals who die
7. the number who survive the infection and become immune or resistant to further infection.

Figure 2–1 shows a schematic relationship between infected and uninfected people for a simple acute infection; all infected individuals either recover from the disease and become immune to it or they die from it. The arrows that connect the boxed groups represent movement of people from one group to an adjacent one.

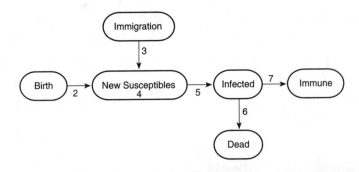

Figure 2–1

Population factors that affect epidemics: 1. Population size; 2. Birth rate; 3. Immigration rate; 4. Number of susceptibles; 5. Transmission rate; 6. Death rate; 7. Immune rate.

This scheme is a simplified representation of the dynamics or ecology of a virus epidemic. It is possible to develop mathematical models to describe or predict an epidemic if the rates of movement through the scheme can be determined. One of the applications of the field of epidemiology (see Chapter 6) is to determine these rates.

The Transmission Rate

The arrow in Figure 2–1 that connects the susceptibles to the infected group is the *transmission rate* of infection. This rate represents the efficiency with which disease is transmitted from an infected person to a susceptible person. This transmission rate has two major components (Figure 2–2). One is the *inherent efficiency* with which a specific virus can infect a susceptible person. The inherent efficiency of a virus is dependent on the biological properties of the virus as well as the route by which the virus enters the susceptible person. For example, influenza virus, like many other respiratory viruses, has a high inherent efficiency of infection and is highly contagious. Respiratory viruses are easily taken up by breathing in aerosols (sneezes), and once influenza virus comes into contact with cells of the respiratory tract, it readily infects them. HIV, on the other hand, actually has a relatively poor inherent infection efficiency, as we shall see later.

The other major component of the transmission rate is the rate at which a susceptible person encounters an infectious person—the *encounter rate*. Each encounter between an infected person and an uninfected person increases the likelihood that an infection will be transmitted.

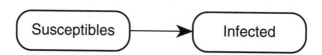

Figure 2–2

Transmission rate of infections has two major components: 1. Inherent efficiency of virus infection; 2. Encounter rate between infected and uninfected.

As we shall see later with the AIDS virus, both of these components of transmission can be changed by altering the behavior of susceptible and infected persons. Behaviors that allow high encounter rates with infected people or that allow more efficient infection will favor the spread of an epidemic. Conversely, changes in behavior that reduce these transmission factors may control the spread of an epidemic.

Population Densities and Infections

Many of the epidemics that have plagued mankind for the last few thousand years would not have had a favorable transmission rate during early human civilization. Early human societies were not urban but consisted of hunter-gatherers who lived in relatively small groups, such as extended families. Such small groups or small populations cannot produce new susceptibles in high enough numbers at any given time to support the continued presence of many epidemic disease microorganisms. An acute disease produces symptoms and makes a person infectious soon after infection. The infected person transmits the disease, dies from the infection, or recovers and becomes immune to subsequent infections. An acute microorganism that strikes such small groups quickly infects all available susceptibles and then dies out.

About 10,000 years ago, the agricultural revolution allowed human populations to become large enough to support epidemics. In other words, the development of human civilization was necessary before epidemics by acute viruses occurred. When the world population became sufficiently large, different patterns of infection also could develop. Epidemic diseases could establish an *endemic pattern*—one in which the disease is always present. Following the initial introduction and spread into a susceptible or naïve population, even a very lethal virus can become endemic. In an endemic disease, the numbers who are actively infected are much lower, but the virus is always present in the population. Endemic viral diseases are often considered childhood diseases because the virus is so common in the population that most individuals encounter it during childhood. Most adults have had the disease and survived. This may be related to the high infant mortality of previous eras (e.g., Europe in the Dark and Middle Ages) and to high infant mortality in some developing countries today. Endemic infectious agents can limit population sizes and result in populations that are relatively unaffected or resistant to the infectious agent as a whole. As we shall see below, this can have major consequences when two previously separated societies encounter each other for the first time.

Chronic Infections

In addition to acute infections, such as measles, there are chronic infections. In *acute infections,* the disease symptoms generally occur quite soon after infection, and the infectious agent is generally eliminated from the individual after the initial disease period. However, some people infected with an acute virus do not develop symptoms (subclinical infections). In a *chronic infection,* the person does not eradicate the infectious agent (often a virus). The virus persists in the infected person and may be produced at low levels. People with chronic infections often do not show symptoms or disease immediately after infection. The differences between acute infection and chronic infection in an infected individual are diagrammed in Figure 2–3. As described earlier, acute infections generally require large populations (with continued new susceptibles) to be maintained. In contrast, chronic infections can sometimes be maintained in small populations. In addition, chronic infections are often more difficult to control because infected and uninfected people may be indistinguishable. As we shall see, the syphilis epidemic was difficult to control partly because it is a chronic infection. Like syphilis, AIDS results from chronic infection.

Controlling Infectious Diseases

Since the beginning of the twentieth century, there has been a steady and dramatic decrease in the number of people who die from infectious diseases, particularly in developed countries. Recently, most developed countries have been free of major lethal contagious diseases. *Antibiotics* can kill bacterial infections after

Acute Infection

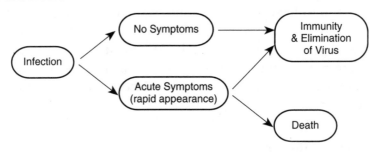

Chronic Infection

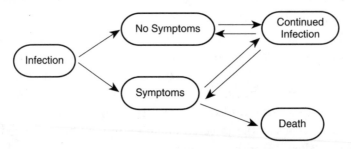

Figure 2–3

Acute versus chronic infection. The consequences of infection of an individual by an acute virus, compared to infection by a chronic virus. The frequencies with which death, immunity, or continued infection occur are different for different viruses.

they start. Viruses pose a different problem: They are difficult to eliminate once they become established. Therefore, viral diseases have been controlled mostly by vaccination (see Chapter 3, p. 40) but occasionally by other measures. A vaccine interrupts the flow of new susceptibles from newborns into the susceptible subpopulation by making young people immune to a virus before they become infected by it (Figure 2–4). If enough (but not necessarily all) susceptibles become immunized, this confers immunity on the population as a whole. This is because the remaining unimmunized but susceptible individuals are unlikely to encounter another infectious individual. It is possible to eliminate some diseases completely from the human population with an effective vaccination program. The smallpox virus, which was responsible

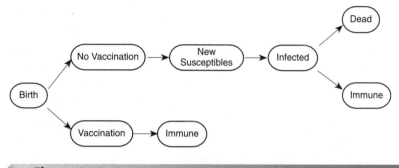

Figure 2–4

Epidemic control by vaccination.

for so much human death in historic times, is now eradicated because of successful worldwide vaccination efforts.

A HISTORY OF EPIDEMICS

The Old World

Even the very earliest historical records document the major impact of epidemics. It is not always clear to us now which infectious agent was causing a particular epidemic in ancient times, but we can often make guesses from the recorded symptoms. The three disease agents that have probably caused most human deaths are smallpox virus, measles virus, and the plague bacterium, *Yersinia pestis*. These three diseases have accounted for hundreds of millions of human deaths over the years and an unfathomable amount of human suffering. Other important epidemic agents include influenza virus, typhoid fever bacterium, yellow fever virus, polio virus, and, more recently, hepatitis viruses. The syphilis bacterium *Treponema pallidum* is of special interest here because of its sexual mode of transmission and its associated social problems.

Many historical accounts make clear reference to a supposed religious or moral reason for a particular epidemic. The transmission of disease itself was often believed to occur through casting of an evil eye. In the Old Testament, for example, Moses brought onto the Egyptians a plague of "sores that break into pustules" due to the sins of the Egyptians. Epidemics were often perceived as punishment due to the wrath of a deity, perhaps for some offense by the entire population. Those who developed a disease were viewed as deserving it. This tendency to link a disease to social stigmatism has persisted throughout history and afflicts people with AIDS today.

The Greek writings are probably the earliest accounts in sufficient detail to allow us to measure the impact of epidemic disease. Aside from malaria, the Greeks were relatively free of most infectious diseases with one important exception. In 430–429 B.C., an epidemic that may have been measles struck Athens with a devastating loss of life. It also resulted in a significant decrease in the size of its armies, and the following year Athens lost a war with Sparta. Thus, this epidemic may have influenced history.

The Roman Empire also suffered massive epidemics in 165 A.D. and again in 251 A.D. Before the 165 A.D. epidemic, the population of the Roman Empire was probably at its peak (about 54 million). After the 165 A.D. and 251 A.D. epidemics, the Roman population did not recover its size until modern times. The first epidemic could have been smallpox and appears to have killed one-third of Rome's population. The 251 A.D. epidemic may have been measles and was equally devastating: There were about 5,000 deaths per day in Rome at its peak. Rome's rural population may have been even more affected. This die-off may have led to the depopulation of agricultural lands and an inability to oppose invasion from the north. A third massive epidemic occurred in 542–543 A.D., probably due to bubonic plague. Soon after this plague, Rome's armies fell to the Visigoth and then to the Moslem armies, and the Dark Age of Europe began. Thus, epidemiological history suggests that infectious diseases may have contributed to the fall of the Roman Empire.

The situation for the Han Chinese society, although more difficult to estimate, appears to have been similar. Massive epidemics in 162 A.D. and again in 310 A.D. may account for much of the population decline in China, which peaked at about 50 million at those times but declined to about 8.9 million by 742 A.D.

In Europe, and probably also in China, measles and small-pox eventually became endemic childhood diseases following these devastating epidemics. In the following millennia, Europe experienced devastating epidemics from the disease known as the *black death*. Black death was a pneumonic form (or lung infection) of plague, which had a very high fatality rate. It probably accounted for up to 100 million deaths in Europe. The worst of these epidemics occurred in 1346. This epidemic appears to have been a *pandemic,* meaning that other continents (China and India) were also involved. The black death recurred in Europe in the 1360s and again in the 1370s. The seemingly arbitrary pattern of death and the massive suffering had dark social consequences for Europe. *Xenophobia,* the fear of foreigners, became common. Violent riots against Jews and Gypsies occurred in numerous cities, because they were blamed as a source of the plague. Self-flagellation became a common practice, and rational theology lost popular acceptance. The situation improved somewhat in the 1400s. Black death became endemic, possibly because of selection for a less virulent plague bacterium; selection for people with greater resistance to the disease also may have occurred. European society was now experiencing most of these acute infectious diseases, especially the viral diseases, as childhood diseases.

The New World

A well-documented example of what happens when a new viral disease enters a naïve population (one that has never encountered the virus) occurred when Cortez went to Mexico and introduced smallpox into the New World. The Aztec Codices (hieroglyphic-like records) tell us that the New World was relatively free of major infectious disease at that time. The population of Mexico was probably 25–30 million, and Mexico City may then have been the most populous city in the world. In 1518, just as the Aztecs drove Cortez from Mexico City, a smallpox epidemic swept though the city, killing the Aztec leaders and decimating the city's population. This epidemic was followed by numerous other diseases that were endemic European childhood diseases but were devastating to the Aztecs. Within 50 years, the population of

Mexico was down to about 1.5 million, or about 5 percent of what it had been at its peak. Furthermore, the fact that the diseases seemed to strike only the Aztecs and not the Spaniards led the Aztecs to believe that the gods favored the Spaniards.

Other American natives fared even worse than the Aztecs: The Native Americans of Baja California and other island tribes became totally extinct. Thus, the main fabric of native American society was utterly destroyed. Mexico began to recover from this population loss only in the 1800s, and only now has Mexico City become the most populous city in the world again. A similar fate was in store for the Pacific island natives, who also suffered huge population losses after encountering European explorers. Thus, throughout human history, infectious diseases have profoundly affected human populations.

MODERN CONCEPTS OF INFECTIOUS DISEASE AND KOCH'S POSTULATES

The germ theory of disease—the idea that a microorganism or "germ" causes an infectious disease—was first proposed in 1546 by Girolamo Fracatoro, a Franciscan monk. However, it was not until the 1840s that H. Henle, a German physician, clarified these concepts and they became accepted among scientists. One of Henle's students, Robert Koch, subsequently proposed four postulates that could be used to prove that an infectious agent causes a disease. This was a milestone in the understanding of infectious disease. *Koch's postulates* state that an organism can be considered to cause a disease if it fulfills the following criteria:

1. The organism is always found in diseased individuals.
2. The organism can be isolated from a diseased individual and grown pure in culture.
3. The pure culture will initiate and reproduce the disease when introduced back into a susceptible host (either man or animal).
4. The organism can be reisolated from that diseased individual.

These postulates allowed scientifically sound assignments of what agents caused specific diseases, and they freed physicians from many superstitions and myths that had historically prevailed.

Actually, by today's standards, Koch's postulates are sometimes too stringent. For example, viruses cannot be grown pure in culture in the absence of cells (see Chapter 4). Also, if two infectious agents cooperate to cause a disease or a particular set of symptoms, it would also be impossible to fulfill Koch's postulates. We shall see that this situation applies to HIV infection and AIDS. In the late 1800s, however, such stringency was necessary.

The timing of the development of Koch's postulates, and of the development of the science of epidemiology, was most fortunate because other changes in society set the stage for the outbreak of another worldwide epidemic. In the late 1800s, steamships brought about relatively rapid world travel. This change had an impact on the ecology of infectious disease by allowing the rapid movement of infected persons who could quickly spread an epidemic. In 1894, another plague pandemic broke out, initially in Burma, then in Hong Kong, then via steamships to all major ports worldwide, including those in the United States. By applying the germ theory of disease and epidemiology, society was able to respond to this threat. The application of Koch's postulates led to the rapid identification and isolation of the causative bacterium, *Yersinia pestis*. Furthermore, intense epidemiological studies identified rats, and more specifically their fleas, as major carriers of the disease. This led to the development of preventive measures to control the spread of the plague, principally by limiting interactions between rats and humans. Except for a further breakout in India, the plague epidemic was stopped. This was an important lesson. There was no cure or vaccine for plague at that time, yet understanding the routes of infection and designing measures based on this understanding to minimize spread of infection averted a pandemic. With the current AIDS epidemic we are in a similar situation, because there is no cure or vaccine. Behavior modification to minimize spread of AIDS virus is currently our only means of controlling the epidemic. However, because AIDS is predominantly a sexually transmitted disease, behavior modification is difficult.

EPIDEMICS IN MODERN TIMES

In the twentieth century, several other epidemics took a toll on humanity. During the great pandemic of 1918, influenza virus killed about 20 million people worldwide and virtually brought World War I to a halt. About 80 percent of American casualties in World War I were caused by influenza, a fact seldom mentioned in most history texts. Influenza continues to cause epidemics and remains a health threat. The major reason is that this virus can mutate rapidly. These mutations lead to changes in the surface structure of the virus that allow the virus to avoid the immune system. As a result, individuals who were previously infected with influenza virus are not protected from the new mutant virus. As we will see later, HIV also has a similar property.

Poliovirus is another recent epidemic disease. This disease appeared as a new viral epidemic in the United States in 1894—much as the AIDS epidemic appeared in 1981. Poliovirus can damage the nervous system and lead to paralysis. In contrast to HIV, which entered North America in the late 1970s (see Chapter 4), poliovirus had been infecting people since early history, but it did not cause documented epidemics until 1894. We now believe that improvements in hygiene and sanitation occurring in more developed societies actually predisposed individuals to the paralytic form of polio by delaying exposure to the virus until they were young adults. Infection of infants, which tends to occur in less developed countries, usually results in a mild nonparalytic gastrointestinal infection. Thus, the people most likely to get paralytic polio were the healthy young adults from the highest socioeconomic classes. This demonstrates the unforeseen effects that changes in social behavior can have on the ecology of an epidemic. Polio had a major impact on the American consciousness, as seen by highly visible national crusades during the first half of the twentieth century (such as the March of Dimes). This underlines the way in which the nature of the victims can influence public perceptions of a disease and society's response to it. In fact, there were about 50,000 total deaths from paralytic polio during the first half of this century. It is interesting to contrast the public response to polio during this time to recent responses to AIDS—

even though more deaths from AIDS occurred in the U.S. in the first ten years of the epidemic.

Syphilis: The Social Problems with a Sexually Transmitted Disease

One epidemic that is hauntingly similar to the AIDS epidemic is syphilis. The parallels are striking. At the time of the syphilis epidemic, scientific investigation of this insidious disease was at the leading edge of medicine and microbiology, as is the current situation with AIDS. The issues raised included public health policy and civil liberties, again as in the AIDS epidemic. And finally, because syphilis is a sexually transmitted disease, patients with that disease were highly stigmatized. A cure for syphilis in infected individuals was developed in 1909, but it was not until the 1940s that the epidemic was finally controlled.

Why did it take so long to control this epidemic? Like AIDS, syphilis can be a long-term and variable disease, with phases in which no symptoms are apparent. Unfortunately, untreated syphilis often eventually leads to death. More important, at that time syphilis was perceived as a social problem—hence the reference to it as a *social disease*. Many blamed the disease on a breakdown of social values and promoted the view that a sexual ethic in which all sex was marital and monogamous would make it impossible to acquire the disease. The initial public health policies to control this epidemic were based on these views. Abstinence from extramarital sexual contact was encouraged, and prostitution was repressed since prostitutes were blamed as the major source of infection of otherwise monogamous males. Immigrants were also blamed for bringing the disease from abroad, even though epidemiological data did not support this view. As many as 20,000 prostitutes were *quarantined* or jailed during World War I. In addition, the Army discouraged the availability of condoms for fear that they might encourage soldiers to engage in extramarital sex. There were also campaigns to stigmatize soldiers who became infected with syphilis by giving them dishonorable discharges. These policies were not based on epidemiological evidence, and they failed to control the epidemic, which actually grew during this period.

It was not until the 1930s that the surgeon general of the United States, Thomas Parren, proposed major changes in the public health approaches to control the syphilis epidemic. These policy changes were ultimately successful but required substantial funding from Congress. The proposals called for the elimination of repressive approaches that discouraged people from participating in programs or seeking treatment. Free and confidential diagnostic and treatment centers were set up throughout the nation. A national educational campaign was begun to educate the public and dispel prevalent misconceptions (even among respected sources) about its transmission. Syphilis is transmitted by sexual contact but not by casual contact. These policies, along with new antibiotics, brought the syphilis epidemic under control in the 1940s.

With the AIDS epidemic, we are dealing with powerful biological drives such as human sexuality and drug addiction. The syphilis epidemic shows us that policies based mainly on abstinence are not very effective in controlling a sexually transmitted disease. Other alterations in behavior are necessary to reduce the transmission of AIDS and bring this epidemic under control. Until a cure or a vaccine against AIDS is developed, changing behavior is our most effective means of controlling the AIDS pandemic.

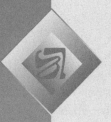

CHAPTER 3
The Immune System

As mentioned in Chapter 1, AIDS results from a viral infection that ultimately disables the immune system. To understand this disease, we need to understand the immune system. This system is an intricate collection of cells and fluids in our body that gives us the ability to fight off infections. HIV, the AIDS virus, specifically affects certain cells of the immune system. Once we know about these cells and what they do, we can see how HIV does its damage. This chapter provides a simplified overview of immunity—many more intricacies and details are known, but the information provided here allows us to understand the basic immunological problems associated with AIDS.

BLOOD

To understand the immune system, we must first consider blood. Blood is a system of circulating cells and fluids that carries out many important functions for the body. These functions include *transport of nutrients and oxygen* to the body tissues, *elimination of waste products and carbon dioxide* from tissues, *wound repair,* and *protection from infection by foreign agents*. Besides cells, the fluid portion of blood contains many different substances and molecules that help carry out these functions. Some examples are sugars that are necessary for energy metabolism in our tissues, and antibodies, which are important in fighting infections. The cell-free fluid portion of blood is referred to as *plasma. Serum* can be obtained from isolated blood by letting it stand and clot; the cells are trapped in the clot and can be removed easily.

Cells and substances of the blood that are responsible for protection from infection make up the *immune system*. The immune system must protect us from a wide variety of infectious agents. These include (in ascending order of complexity):

Viruses. These are very small subcellular agents (see Chapter 4).

Bacteria. These are small, single-cell microorganisms, which have relatively simple genetic material. Typhoid fever and tuberculosis are caused by bacteria.

Protozoa. These are single-cell microorganisms that contain more complicated genetic structures. Amoebas and Giardia are examples of protozoa.

Fungi. These are more complex microorganisms that may exist as single cells, or they may be organized into simple multicellular organisms. Examples are yeasts and molds.

Multicellular parasites. These can be relatively large organisms, such as roundworms and tapeworms.

In addition, the immune system is also important in fighting cancer.

Blood is carried throughout the body by a series of blood vessels that make up the *circulatory system* (Figure 3–1). The heart is the pump for the circulatory system, and it moves blood through the blood vessels by its rhythmic muscular contractions. There are three kinds of blood vessels: *arteries*, which carry blood away from the heart to the body tissues; *veins*, which carry blood back to the heart from the tissues; and *capillaries*. Capillaries are very thin-walled blood vessels in the tissues that connect the arteries with the veins, and they allow exchange of oxygen, nutrients, and wastes between the blood and tissues. Some kinds of blood cells (such as the white blood cells called *monocytes* and *lymphocytes*) can also pass through these thin walls from the blood into the tissues as well. The lungs are another important part of the circulatory system—this is where the exchange of oxygen and carbon dioxide between the blood and the air we breathe takes place.

The cells in the blood have limited life spans—ranging from one or two days to several weeks, depending on the cell type. This means that they must be continually replenished. They are replenished from *stem cells* located in the bone marrow. These stem cells have the capacity to divide and make more of themselves and to differentiate and mature into blood cells of all types (Figure 3–2). During the differentiation process, the stem cells first develop into *committed precursors,* which can either divide or differentiate into mature blood cells of a particular kind. This process goes on throughout life and, if interrupted, results in very serious health problems.

When stem cells and committed precursors divide or differentiate, they require the presence of *growth factors* to carry out

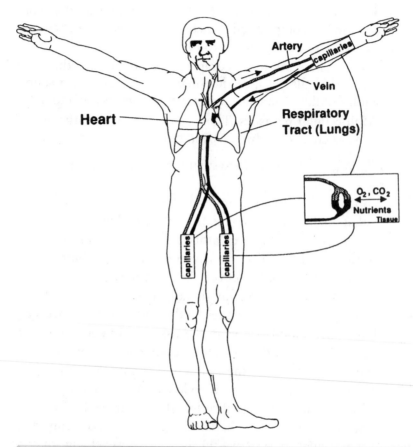

Figure 3–1

The circulatory system.

these processes. Different growth factors stimulate particular kinds of blood cells, and these growth factors play important roles in regulating the orderly growth and replenishment of all blood cells. For example, interleukin 2 (IL-2) is a growth factor that is required by blood cells called T-lymphocytes, which are discussed later.

Cells of the Blood

Let us now look at the different kinds of cells present in blood. These cells are shown in Figure 3–3. Blood cells are divided into *red blood cells* and *white blood cells*. There are a lot of red blood

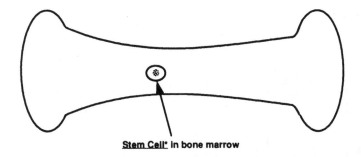

Stem Cell* in bone marrow

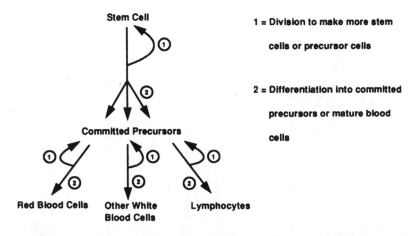

Figure 3–2

Growth and maturation of blood cells.

cells, but they are a single cell type; the white blood cells are fewer in number, but they are made up of many cell types.

Red Blood Cells

Red blood cells or *erythrocytes* are responsible for carrying oxygen to the tissues and carbon dioxide away from them. They contain a protein called *hemoglobin* that binds and carries the oxygen and carbon dioxide within them. Hemoglobin gives red blood cells their characteristic red color. All the other blood cells are called white blood cells, since they lack hemoglobin.

White Blood Cells

White blood cells or *leukocytes* are of several different types. *Megakaryocytes* are very large blood cells that bud off subcellular

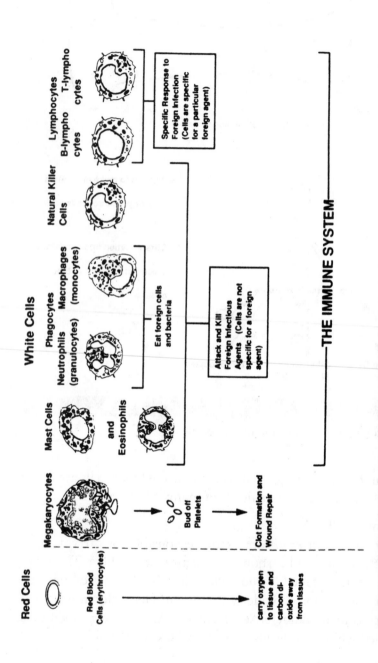

Figure 3-3

Cells of the blood.

bind directly and inhibit the function of infectious agents such as viruses. These are called *neutralizing antibodies.*

T-lymphocytes (or T-cells) make proteins called *receptors* that are similar to antibodies in that these proteins recognize specific antigens. However, T-lymphocytes do not release their receptors but hold them on their cell surfaces. As a result, the T-lymphocytes themselves specifically recognize and bind to foreign antigens.

The two major kinds of T-lymphocytes are *cytotoxic or killer T-cells* (T_{killer}) and *helper T-cells* (T_{helper}). T_{killer} cells directly bind to cells carrying a foreign antigen. Once they bind to them, they attack and kill those cells, thus eliminating them from the body. T_{helper} cells, on the other hand, do not kill cells. Instead, they interact with B-lymphocytes or T_{killer} lymphocytes and help them respond to antigens (more about this later). In addition to the receptors, T_{killer} and T_{helper} cells each have characteristic proteins on their surfaces: the *CD8* protein is present on T_{killer} cells, and the *CD4* protein is present on T_{helper} cells (Figure 3–5). Simple tests

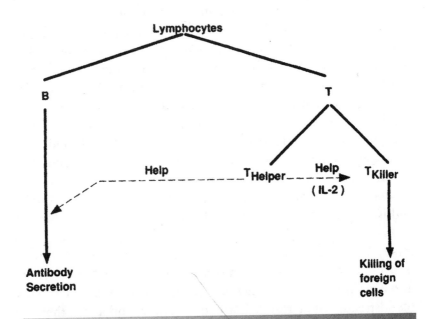

Figure 3–5

Kinds of lymphocytes.

have been devised for the CD4 and CD8 proteins, and they can be used to identify and count T_{killer} and T_{helper} lymphocytes.

T-lymphocytes get their name from the fact that their maturation depends on passage through the thymus gland. The thymus is a butterfly-shaped gland that lies over the heart.

Natural killer cells are cells that resemble T-lymphocytes in many physical properties, although they also show some differences. These cells attack virus-infected cells and tumor cells and kill them. Natural killer cells exist in normal individuals who have not previously encountered the infectious agent or cancer—this is different from the situation for B- and T-lymphocytes, as we shall see below. Furthermore, individual natural killer cells are not specific for the cells they attack, which also distinguishes them from B- and T-lymphocytes (see below).

THE LYMPHATIC CIRCULATION

Lymphocytes (both B-cells and T-cells) circulate through the blood vessels and also through a second circulatory system, the *lymphatic circulation*. The lymphatic circulation is made up of *lymph channels* in our tissues, which drain lymph fluid from the tissues into structures called *lymph nodes* (Figure 3–6). The lymph nodes contain B-lymphocytes and T-lymphocytes, which can respond to foreign antigens during infections. As an example, suppose a tissue becomes infected with a virus. Pieces of virus or whole virus particles will be transported in the lymph fluid down the lymph channels to the lymph node. In the lymph node, the virus may be recognized as an antigen by B- or T-lymphocytes, which respond by secreting antibodies specific for the virus or by producing T-lymphocytes specific for the virus. These antibodies and lymphocytes are then drained from the lymph node through another lymph channel, which joins other lymph channels from other parts of the tissue. Ultimately, fluid from lymph nodes all over the body is collected in a series of lymph vessels that empty into a main vessel called the *thoracic duct,* which empties into the bloodstream. As a result, antibodies and lymphocytes that are produced in response to an infection at one site or tissue will be distributed by the bloodstream throughout the body.

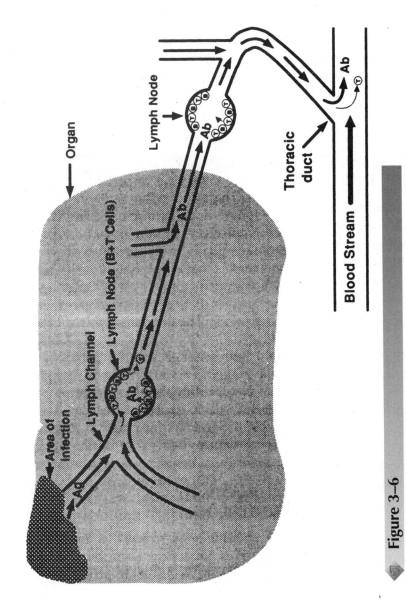

Figure 3–6

The lymphatic circulation.

During infections, the lymph nodes near the site of the infection frequently become enlarged. This is because the lymphocytes in these lymph nodes are dividing rapidly and producing large amounts of antibodies and cells to fight the infectious agent. You may have noticed swollen glands in your neck if you get a respiratory infection. This is an example of this process. The spleen is another organ in the body that has many of the same cells that a lymph node has. These spleen cells carry out functions similar to those of the lymph nodes.

B-CELLS AND HUMORAL IMMUNITY: THE GENERATION OF ANTIBODIES

Let us now look at how B-lymphocytes respond to a foreign antigen by making antibodies. This part of the immune system is referred to as *humoral immunity,* since it results in production of antibodies which circulate in the bloodstream. *Humor* is derived from the Latin word for fluid.

Antibodies

An antibody molecule is made up of four proteins that are bound together: Two of these proteins are identical and are called *heavy chains*; the other two are also identical and are called *light chains*. A protein is a linear chain of building-block molecules called *amino acids*—much like beads on a string. There are 20 possible amino acids, and the nature of a protein is determined by the particular sequence of the amino acids it contains (Figure 3–7). In the case of antibodies, the two heavy chain proteins are larger than the two light chain proteins. These proteins are held together by chemical bonding into a Y-shaped molecule, as shown in Figure 3–8. Each antibody molecule is specific for one particular antigen, and this specificity is determined by the sequence of amino acids in the light and heavy chains. If several different antibodies with different specificities are compared, certain regions of the light and heavy chains are very similar for the different antibodies. These regions are referred to as *constant re-*

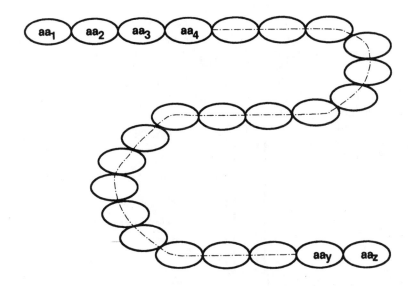

aa1=amino acid number 1 in the protein chain

aa2=amino acid number 2 in the protein chain

etc.

Figure 3–7

Protein structure.

gions or C-regions. Other parts of the light and heavy chain proteins are different for each different antibody in terms of the amino acid building-block sequence. These parts are called the *variable regions* or V-regions. The protein sequences of the variable regions determine which antigen the antibody binds to. An antibody fits its antigen as a key fits only its own lock. Once an antibody is bound to its proper antigen, the C-regions then signal other parts of the immune system to attack—for instance, phagocytosis by a neutrophil or macrophage (see Figure 3–4).

One important feature of the humoral immune system is that *each B-lymphocyte makes only one type of antibody,* with a single specificity for an antigen. Thus, each B-lymphocyte is specific for one antigen.

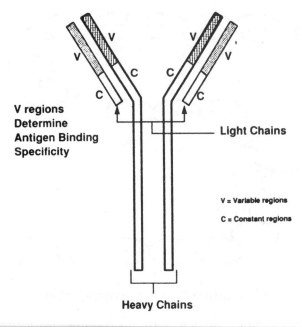

**V regions
Determine
Antigen Binding
Specificity**

Light Chains

V = Variable regions

C = Constant regions

Heavy Chains

Figure 3–8

Structure of an antibody molecule.

How Does the Immune System Respond to New Antigens?

During our lives, the number of different infectious agents and antigens that we might encounter is infinite. To protect us from disease, the immune system must be able to respond to each new antigen on demand by making new antibodies that recognize it. On the other hand, it is impossible for the immune system to anticipate all possible antigens and continually make all possible antibodies that might be required all the time. This would be much too costly in terms of energy and genetic material. To solve this dilemma, the immune system uses two processes: generation of antibody gene diversity by DNA rearrangement and clonal selection.

Generation of Antibody Gene Diversity by DNA Rearrangement

The genetic information for the antibody proteins is contained within DNA in our chromosomes. *DNA is a long molecule made

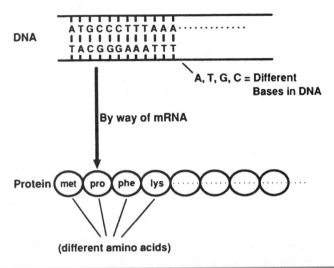

DNA

ATGCCCTTTAAA ············

TACGGGAAATTT

A, T, G, C = Different Bases in DNA

By way of mRNA

Protein met pro phe lys ···· ··· ···· ···

(different amino acids)

Figure 3–9

How genetic information in DNA is converted into protein.

up of two strands wound around each other. Each strand is a chain made up of building blocks called *nucleotides*, which contain four possible *bases* (adenine or A, cytosine or C, thymine or T, and guanosine or G). The exact order of bases in a DNA molecule specifies the order of amino acid building blocks in the corresponding protein, as shown in Figure 3–9. The sequence of DNA bases that specifies one protein is referred to as a *gene*. Each of our chromosomes contains many thousands of genes along its DNA molecule. We inherit two sets of DNA molecules in the form of chromosomes—one set from our mother and one set from our father. The DNA content of most of the cells in the body is the same—different kinds of cells make different kinds of proteins by selecting which genes will be expressed by way of messenger RNA (see Chapter 4) for synthesis into protein. However, antibody-producing B-lymphocytes are an exception, at least as far as the region of the chromosome that specifies antibody proteins is concerned.

It is important to remember that each mature B-lymphocyte produces only one kind of antibody. Thus, each B-lymphocyte makes one kind of heavy chain protein and one kind of light chain. All the cells in the body actually contain multiple copies of the genes for variable regions of the heavy and light chain proteins. For the heavy chains, the variable region is actually expressed from three sets of genes called *V-genes, D-genes,* and *J-genes.* There are about 200 different V-genes, about 50 different D-genes, and about 10 different J-genes. During development and maturation of a B-lymphocyte, the DNA in the chromosomes surrounding the antibody genes is rearranged (Figure 3–10). As a result of the rearrangement, one V-gene is brought together with one D- and one J-gene, and this combination is next to the gene for the constant region. The intervening V, D, and J DNA sequences are deleted. This VDJ combination is expressed along with the constant region gene to give the heavy chain protein. Light chain protein also results from a similar DNA rearrangement process, except that the variable region is specified by only two sets of multiple genes, V-genes and J-genes.

The DNA rearrangements of the antibody genes (VDJ for heavy chain and VJ for light chains) in any individual developing B-lymphocyte are *randomly selected* from the various possible V-, D- and J-genes. Thus, the total number of possible VDJ combinations for the heavy chains in a B-lymphocyte is the *product* of the number of V-genes times the number of D-genes, times the number of J-genes (200 V-genes × 50 D-genes × 10 J-genes = 100,000 combinations for the variable region). Similarly, the total possible VJ combinations for light chain proteins is the product of the

Before DNA Rearrangement

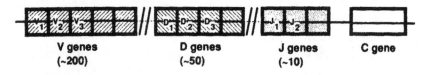

| V genes (~200) | D genes (~50) | J genes (~10) | C gene |

After DNA Rearrangement

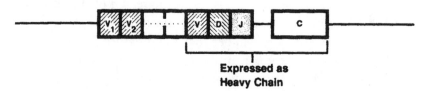

Expressed as
Heavy Chain

Figure 3–10

DNA rearrangement for expression of antibodies.

number of light chain V-genes times the number of light chain J-genes. Since each B-lymphocyte produces antibody containing one heavy chain and one light chain, the total number of possible antibodies a B-lymphocyte can make is the product of the possible kinds of heavy chain proteins times the possible kinds of light chain proteins. Thus, the number of possible antibodies that a B-lymphocyte can make is many millions.

Another process also takes place during B-lymphocyte maturation in addition to the DNA rearrangement of the antibody genes. Individual DNA bases in the genes for the variable regions may be changed or added. These changes will further alter the amino acid sequences of the variable regions for the light and heavy chain proteins. Since these changes also occur on a random basis, they *further increase* the number of kinds of variable regions on the antibody proteins. In practice, the number of possible kinds of antibody proteins that can be made is almost limitless.

Clonal Selection

In a normal, uninfected individual, many different B-lymphocytes have each carried out the DNA rearrangements of their antibody genes, and more mature every day. Initially, these B-lymphocytes express their specific antibodies on their outer surfaces, but they do not secrete antibody and they do not divide. However, if a particular B-lymphocyte recognizes an antigen that binds to its specific antibody (for instance, a protein from an infecting virus), it receives a *signal for activation*. Other B-lymphocytes that are present but that have not bound an antigen do not receive the activation signal. If the B-lymphocyte that has bound an antigen also receives a *second signal* (discussed later), it becomes *fully activated* (Figure 3–11). A fully activated B-lymphocyte does two things: It *divides rapidly* and generates more activated B-cells that make the same antibody, and these activated B-cells all *secrete the specific antibody* into the extracellular space (for instance, the lymph or blood). The result of this process is the production of large amounts of antibody specific for the antigen.

The Primary Immune Response

The primary immune response occurs when the immune system encounters an antigen for the first time, as shown in Figure 3–12.

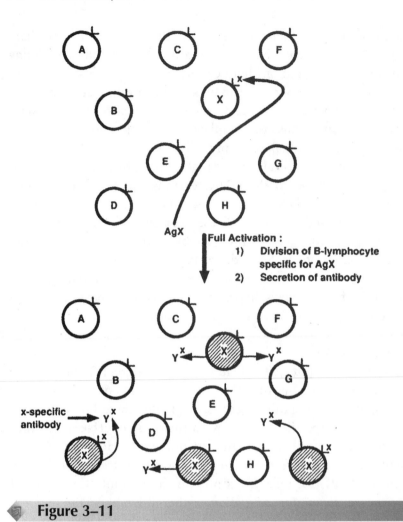

Figure 3–11

Clonal selection of B-lymphocytes.

For several days after an antigen is encountered, there are no antibodies for the antigen in the bloodstream. This lag period can last for as little as 10 days or as much as several weeks. During the lag period, B-lymphocytes are being primed with antigen and activated to divide and produce antibody. Eventually, antibodies specific for the antigen begin to appear in the bloodstream and increase until they reach a plateau level. Then, if the antigen is eliminated, the antibody level slowly falls until it returns to an undetectable (or barely detectable) level.

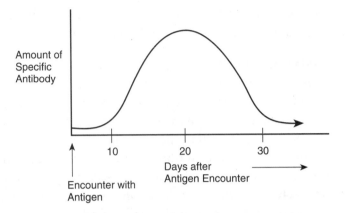

Figure 3–12

The primary immune response.

In terms of infectious agents such as viruses and bacteria, the lag period during the primary immune response is very important. During this period, no antibodies against the microorganism are being produced. Thus, the individual is susceptible to continued infection during this period—the immune system will begin to fight most efficiently only after antibodies are produced. This window of vulnerability is particularly critical for virus infections, since it is often very difficult to eliminate them once they have become established (see Chapter 4, p. 56).

During the primary immune response, many different B-lymphocytes become primed and activated to produce antibodies. For instance, in the case of a virus infection, B-lymphocytes that make antibodies specific for different virus proteins are activated. Furthermore, different B-lymphocytes may make antibodies for different parts of a single virus protein. All these B-lymphocytes contribute to the mixture of antibodies that makes up the immune response.

As the primary immune response progresses, the quality of the antibodies also improves. Those antibodies whose variable regions bind most tightly to the antigen become predominant. In addition, the nature of the constant regions of the antibody molecules changes. This leads to more efficient signaling by the antibodies to other cells of the immune system (such as phagocytes) for attack and destruction of the foreign cell or microorganism.

The Secondary Immune Response

A *secondary immune response* occurs in individuals who have previously raised an immunological reaction against a particular antigen—for instance, someone who has recovered from an infection and then later encounters the same infectious agent. In this case, the levels of specific antibodies rise very rapidly, almost without a lag (Figure 3–13). The levels of specific antibody also fall more slowly than after the primary immune response. In addition, the antibodies are of the high-quality kind, which bind antigen tightly and efficiently signal to other immune cells for attack. Thus the immune system is said to have *immunological memory*—the ability to respond rapidly and efficiently to an antigen that has been encountered previously.

Vaccines

The nature of the primary and secondary immune responses and immunological memory have led to development of *vaccines* and *vaccination* for controlling infections. The principle is to preexpose an individual to part of an infectious agent that cannot cause disease (the vaccine) and to induce production of antibodies against that agent. Repeated injections during the initial immunization often induce the production of high-quality antibodies. After the initial immunization, booster injections at regular intervals stimulate the immunological memory and maintain circulating antibodies for the infectious agent. These antibodies prevent the infectious agent from establishing itself in a vaccinated individual.

Tolerance

Normal tissues in our bodies contain many molecules that could possibly serve as antigens for our own immune systems. It would be very detrimental to our health if our immune systems attacked our own tissues. Indeed, there are immunological disorders called *autoimmune diseases* that consist of immunological attack of an individual's own tissue (for instance, rheumatoid arthritis). In

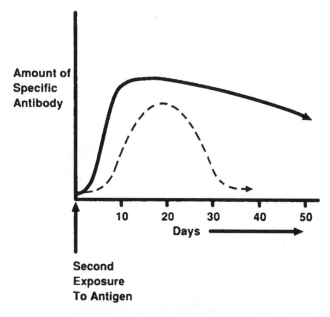

Amount of Specific Antibody

10   20   30   40   50

Days

Second Exposure To Antigen

Figure 3–13

The secondary immune response (——) compared with a primary immune response (------).

normal individuals, the immune system distinguishes between *self* and *non-self*. This is achieved by the development of *tolerance* toward normal tissues. For the most part, this is accomplished by elimination during early development of B- and T-lymphocytes that recognize normal tissues. Since these self-specific lymphocytes are absent, no immunological response toward normal tissue will occur. In addition, other T-lymphocytes provide a second line of defense, should some self-specific lymphocytes avoid elimination. These lymphocytes are called $T_{suppressor}$ lymphocytes, and they prevent B-lymphoctes or T_{helper} lymphocytes specific for self-antigens from maturing. $T_{suppressor}$ lymphocytes have CD8 protein on their surfaces, like T_{killer} lymphocytes.

A Summary of the Humoral Immune System

To summarize the humoral immune system:

1. B-lymphocytes make antibody molecules, and each B-cell makes only one kind of antibody.

2. The immune response is based on

    a. generation of many B-lymphocytes with different antibody specificities by DNA rearrangement and mutation within the antibody genes, and

    b. clonal expansion of B-cells that recognize their specific antigen when infection occurs.

3. Antibodies fight infections by

    a. direct neutralization of viruses,

    b. binding to targets and signaling phagocytes or other white blood cells to attack, or

    c. binding to target cells and signaling for other host defense mechanisms.

T-Cells and Cell-Mediated Immunity

As described above, T-cells make *T-cell antigen receptors* that resemble antibodies made by B-cells. As with an antibody, the T-cell receptor variable region determines its specificity toward an antigen. Also like B-lymphocytes, each T-lymphocyte makes only one kind of T-cell antigen receptor. Thus, each T-lymphocyte is specific for a particular antigen. As described above, T-lymphocytes do not release their receptors; instead, the receptors are anchored in the cell surface, and the variable regions project outside. As a result, T-lymphocytes will bind to cells expressing antigen by way of their T-cell antigen receptor. T-lymphocytes represent *cell-mediated immunity*, since the cells themselves specifically bind with antigens. This contrasts with humoral immunity, in which antibodies released from B-lymphocytes carry out the antigen binding.

T$_{killer}$ Lymphocytes

T$_{killer}$ lymphocytes (also called cytotoxic T-lymphocytes) bind cells carrying a foreign antigen and directly kill those cells. Once they have carried out this killing, they release from the target cell, which has been destroyed, and can bind and kill other cells. An example of such an interaction is shown in Figure 3–14. Some examples of cells that T$_{killer}$ cells attack include:

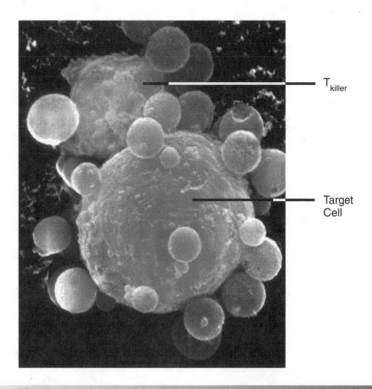

T_{killer}

Target
Cell

Figure 3–14

T_{killer} lymphocyte killing a target cell (the largest cell) (electron microscope picture). *(Courtesy Dr. Andrejs Liepins/Science Photo Library)*

1. *Virus-infected cells.* Most cells infected with viruses express some of the viral proteins (or parts of them) on their outer surfaces. These viral proteins can be recognized as foreign antigens and bind T_{killer} lymphocytes. As a result, the virus-infected cells are killed.

2. *Tumor cells.* When cancers develop, they often express abnormal proteins on their outer surfaces. These abnormal proteins can also provoke an immune response by T-lymphocytes, which results in immunological attack on the tumor cells. In fact, the immune system is an important part of our natural defense against cancer. During our lives, probably many cells in our bodies begin to develop into tumors, but the cell-mediated immune system eliminates them before they can grow very much. This is called *immunological surveillance*. This is

also important in AIDS because, as we shall see, failure of the immune system can result in development of cancers. In addition to T-lymphocytes, natural killer cells (discussed earlier) are also very important in immunological surveillance.

3. *Tissue Rejection.* When tissue from an unrelated individual is introduced into another person, the cell-mediated immune system will generally raise a strong response and kill the transplanted tissue. This is because cell surface proteins called *histocompatibility antigens* generally differ from individual to individual. This is a major problem for medical procedures such as skin grafting and organ transplantation. When tissue with different histocompatibility antigens is transplanted into an individual, a strong cell-mediated immune response against these antigens occurs, and the transplanted tissue is destroyed. In the case of organ transplantation, donors and recipients must be carefully matched

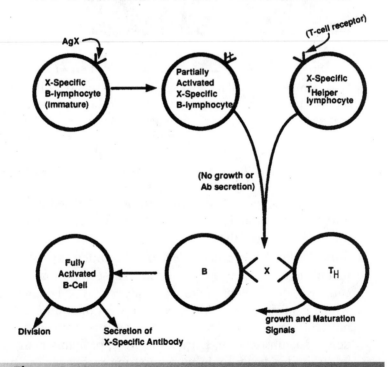

Figure 3–15

The role of T_{helper} cells in B-lymphocyte activation.

for histocompatibility antigens to avoid rejection of the donor organ. Even then, the recipients must take immunosuppressive drugs permanently to avoid rejection of the donated organ.

T_{helper} Lymphocytes

T_{helper} lymphocytes play a central role in both humoral and cell-mediated immunity. In *humoral immunity,* they provide the second signal necessary for a B-lymphocyte that has bound antigen to divide and secrete antibodies (see Figure 3–11). In fact, in order for a B-lymphocyte that has bound antigen to become fully activated, a T_{helper} lymphocyte with the *same antigenic specificity* must bind the antigen as well, as shown in Figure 3–15. Once the

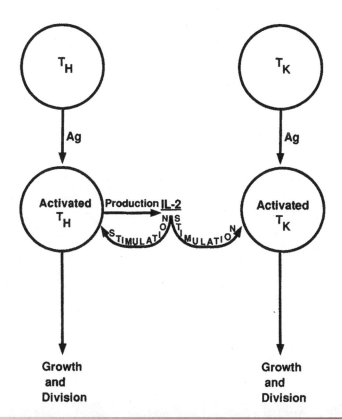

Figure 3–16

T_{helper} cells in cell-mediated immunity.

specific T_{helper} lymphocyte is bound to the B-lymphocyte by way of the antigen, it provides growth and maturation signals to the B-cell, leading to growth and antibody production. If a T_{helper} lymphocyte of the same antigen specificity as the B-lymphocyte is absent, the B-lymphocyte will not complete maturation, even if it has bound antigen.

T_{helper} cells also play an important role in *cell-mediated* immunity. When T-lymphocytes (either T_{helper} or T_{killer}) bind antigen, they become activated to divide. This results in increased numbers of specific T-lymphocytes to fight the foreign infectious agent. However, as for many blood cells, T-lymphocytes also need a growth factor to divide (as discussed above). For T-lymphocytes that have bound antigen, the required growth factor is one called *interleukin 2* or *IL-2*. It turns out that T_{helper} lymphocytes produce and secrete IL-2 when they are activated by antigen binding (Figure 3–16). Thus, the T_{helper} lymphocytes can stimulate themselves to divide after they bind antigen. On the other hand, most T_{killer} cells do not produce IL-2 even after they bind antigen. They

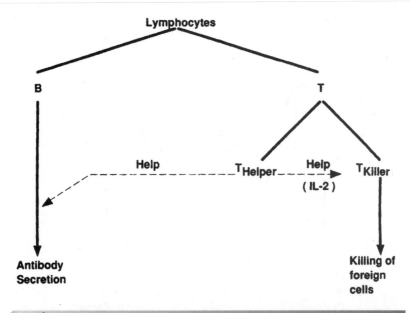

Figure 3–17

The central role of T_{helper} lymphocytes.

generally rely on IL-2 secreted by neighboring T_{helper} cells to divide. In this case, the neighboring T_{helper} cell that produces the IL-2 does not have to be specific for the same antigen as the T_{killer} cell it helps. Thus, if T_{helper} lymphocytes are absent, T_{killer} cells cannot divide even if they have bound their specific antigens.

In summary, T_{helper} lymphocytes play a central role in both humoral and cell-mediated immunity, as illustrated in Figure 3–17. As we shall see in the next chapter, the major problem in AIDS is that the causative agent HIV specifically infects and kills T_{helper} lymphocytes. This causes a failure of both the humoral immune system and cell-mediated immunity. As a result, immunological protection against infectious agents is impaired or cancer develops.

CHAPTER 4
Virology and Human Immunodeficiency Virus

In this chapter, we first look at viruses in general, then retroviruses, and then HIV, the virus that causes AIDS, in particular. We will also see how the HIV antibody test (used for screening for HIV infection) works and what it tells us. We will then consider the basis of action of the drug azidothymidine (AZT) and of protease inhibitors, which are currently used as antiviral treatments for HIV infection.

A GENERAL INTRODUCTION TO VIRUSES

Let's first consider viruses in a general sense. There are many different kinds of viruses, and many of them cause disease. Individual viruses may differ in their exact composition and mechanism for growth, but all viruses have some common properties.

What Are Viruses?

Viruses are among the simplest life forms. Here are some of the common features of viruses:

1. **Viruses** *are obligate intracellular parasites.* This means that viruses cannot replicate and make more of themselves outside cells. In fact, a pure preparation of virus particles will not grow. In the case of humans, this means that viruses must replicate in some tissue or cell type in our bodies.

2. *Virus particles consist of the following components* (see Figure 4–1):

   a. *Genetic material.* Viruses carry genetic material in the form of *nucleic acids.* For some viruses, the nucleic acid is DNA, the same as the genetic material of the cells in our bodies. For other viruses, the nucleic acid is *RNA,* which is related chemically to DNA (discussed later). *The genetic material of a virus specifies virus proteins.* These virus proteins may be *structural proteins* that make up the virus particles, *enzymes* that help carry out biochemical processes necessary for virus growth, or *regulatory proteins.* Some viral regulatory proteins are used by the virus to select expression of particular virus genes at dif-

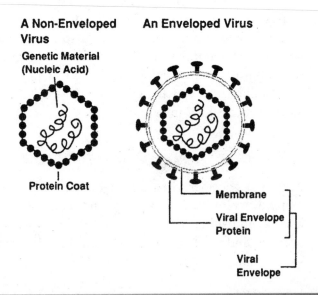

A Non-Enveloped Virus

Genetic Material (Nucleic Acid)

Protein Coat

An Enveloped Virus

Membrane

Viral Envelope Protein

Viral Envelope

Figure 4–1

Structure of a typical virus.

ferent times or under different conditions. Other viral regulatory proteins may be used by the virus to help it take over the cell and convert it into an efficient factory for producing the virus.

b. *A system for protecting the genetic material and introducing it into a cell.* Viruses must protect their genetic material when they leave one cell and move to another—either within tissues of an infected individual or from an infected individual to an uninfected one. Naked DNA or RNA is quite fragile and vulnerable to attack by numerous agents. Thus, viruses carry genes that direct production of a *protein coat* that surrounds the genetic material. In addition, some (but not all) viruses direct synthesis of a *viral envelope* that surrounds the virus's genetic information and protein coat. Viral envelopes resemble the membranes that make up the outer surfaces of our cells. These membranes contain proteins that are virus specified. For viruses that contain envelopes, the envelope proteins are very important for the initial phases of infection, since they are exposed on the outside of the virus particle.

3. *Viruses are dependent on cells for:*

a. *Energy metabolism.* Energy is required for most biochemical processes to take place. In the case of viruses, such processes include those responsible for production of the virus's proteins and genetic material. However, viruses themselves do not carry the machinery necessary for generating energy. Instead, they rely on the machinery of the cells they infect.

b. *Protein synthesis.* Proteins are synthesized in cells by a complex system of molecules and subcellular particles, using instructions from the genetic material. Again, viruses carry the genetic instructions but do not carry the machinery for synthesis of proteins. They depend on the cell protein synthesis machinery.

c. *Nucleic acid synthesis.* Many viruses may also depend on the cell machinery for synthesis of virus-specific nucleic acids. These nucleic acids may be used for expression of viral proteins (mRNA, discussed later), or they may be the virus's genetic information itself.

How Does a Virus Infect a Host?

For a virus to infect an individual, it must come into contact with a susceptible cell. It is important to remember that most of the human body is covered with skin, which protects us from infection: Skin is quite tough, and the outer layers of skin cells are actually dead. Thus, most viruses cannot infect and grow in cells of the outer layers of the skin. These are some of the important routes that viruses use to enter the body (Figure 4–2):

> *The respiratory tract:* Viruses can be carried into the respiratory tract through the air we breathe. Once they are brought into the body by this route, they can infect cells in any part of the respiratory tract, including the nose, windpipe,

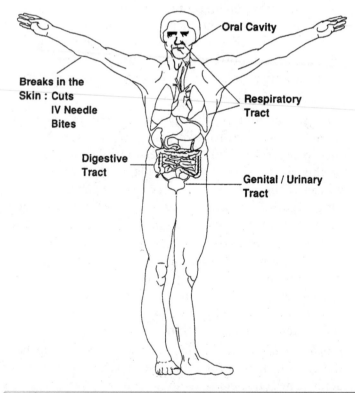

Figure 4–2

Routes of entry for viruses.

bronchial tubes, and lungs. Examples of viruses that infect the respiratory tract are influenza and the common cold.

The oral cavity and digestive tract: If viruses are taken in with food or water, they can potentially infect cells of the mouth and other parts of the digestive system, including the large and small intestines. One form of liver inflammation, or hepatitis (infectious or type A hepatitis), is an example of this category, as are various diarrheas.

The anal/genital tract: During sexual intercourse, it is possible to introduce viruses into the female or male anal/genital tract from an infected partner. Such infections are classified as venereal diseases. If sexual intercourse involves anal penetration, it is possible to introduce viruses into the anus, rectum, and lower intestines by this route as well. Genital herpes virus is an example of an infection of the genital tract. As we shall see, genital tract infection is an important route for HIV and AIDS.

Breaks in the skin: If the protective layer of skin is broken by a cut or scratch, then viruses may be able to enter directly into tissues or the bloodstream. *Bites from animals or insects* also fall into this category. For example, rabies is spread by bites from infected animals such as dogs or squirrels, and yellow fever is spread by bites from infected mosquitoes. *Transfusions* and *injection drug use* are other examples of infection through breaks in the skin. In these cases, viruses that contaminate blood or blood products can be introduced into individuals during transfusions with blood or blood products or during injection drug use involving shared needles. For example, another form of hepatitis, hepatitis B, can be spread by injection drug use (as well as sexual contact). Injection drug use (and, originally, transfusions) is another important route of infection for HIV.

It is important to remember that any individual type of virus will use some but not all of these routes of infection. A key to controlling viral infections is understanding the particular routes of spread the virus of interest uses. We shall see how this is determined in Chapter 6. After a virus has entered an individual and established infection at a *primary site*, the infection can spread to *secondary sites* in the body as well. Disease symptoms may result from infection at the primary site, the secondary sites, or both.

A Typical Virus Infection Cycle

Let's look at what happens if a purified virus preparation is used to infect some susceptible cells in the laboratory. A typical result is shown in Figure 4–3. If the amount of infectious virus is measured over a period of time, it is seen to fall after an initial lag period, remain low for a period of time, and then rise to even higher levels. The period during which the amount of infectious virus is low is referred to as the *eclipse* period. The virus infection cycle can be divided into several events:

1. *Adsorption (binding)* of the virus to the cell. When a virus infects, it must first bind to the cell. This binding is a very specific interaction between the virus particle and some protein (or other molecule) on the cell surface. This protein is referred to as the virus *receptor*. At first, it might seem strange that cells have receptors for viruses, since this would seem to be disadvantageous to the uninfected host. How-

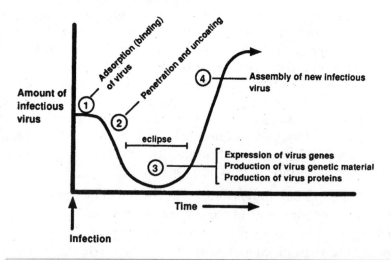

Figure 4–3

A typical virus infection cycle within a cell.

ever, this is due to the fact that viruses have evolved so that they are able to bind to a protein that is normally present on the uninfected cell. The distribution of the receptor protein among different cells in the body influences the kinds of cells that the virus can infect. We will see that this is an important consideration for HIV infection and development of AIDS.

2. *Penetration* of the virus into the cell and *uncoating* of the viral genetic material. Once the virus particles have bound to the surface of the cell by attaching to a receptor protein, they are brought into the cell. This penetration process is an active one that requires expenditure of energy by the cell. Once the virus particle has been taken into the cell, its protective protein coat is removed, exposing the viral genetic material. The genetic material is now ready to be expressed. This uncoating of the virus accounts for the drop in infectious virus assayed because the uncoated virus cannot withstand the assay conditions.

3. *Expression of the viral genetic material.* This occurs during the eclipse period, when the amount of infectious virus in the culture appears low. Several events take place during the eclipse phase:

   a. *Organization of the infected cell for virus expression.* The cell machinery may be altered to favor efficient expression of virus genes. This often occurs at the expense of the cell's own metabolic processes and may ultimately lead to death of the infected cell.

   b. *Replication of the viral genetic material.* The virus programs the machinery necessary to generate more copies of its own genetic material. In some cases, this may rely on machinery from the uninfected cell, but in other cases, the virus may specify proteins that are necessary for the process.

   c. *Synthesis of proteins for virus particles.* Proteins that make up the virus coat, as well as those in the viral envelope, are synthesized from instructions in the viral genetic information. Once these proteins are synthesized, all the components necessary for formation of a new virus particle are present within the infected cell.

4. *Assembly of virus particles and release* from the cell. Virus particles are assembled in the infected cell from the new genetic material and viral proteins. As this occurs, the amount of infectious virus in the culture increases and surpasses that at the start of the infection. Typically, an infected cell releases hundreds or thousands of new virus particles, which can spread to infect other cells.

Depending on the virus, there are different fates for an infected cell. For many viruses, the infected cell is killed (or lysed) at the end of the infection. These viruses are called *lytic*. Other viruses do not kill the infected cell, but they establish a persistent or carrier state in which the cell survives and continually produces virus particles. These viruses are called *nonlytic*. Some viruses can also establish a state called *latency* in cells. In these situations, the virus's genetic material remains hidden in the cell, but no virus is produced. At a later time, the latent virus can become *reactivated*, and the cell will begin to produce infectious virus particles again, as in the case of cold sores caused by a herpes virus. As we shall see, all these fates probably play an important role in HIV infection and the development of AIDS.

How Do We Treat Viral Infections?

When virus infections become established, they are very difficult to treat. This contrasts with the wide variety of antibiotics available to treat infections by other microorganisms such as bacteria and fungi. Antibiotics take advantage of the fact that there are differences in some of the biochemical machinery of these very simple microorganisms compared to highly developed organisms such as humans. These antibiotics specifically inhibit processes carried out by the bacteria or fungi, but they do not affect similar processes in higher organisms. For instance, the antibiotic streptomycin inhibits the intracellular machinery used to make proteins in bacteria but not in humans. Unfortunately, since viruses rely on the cell to carry out most of their metabolic processes, it is difficult to find drugs similar to classical antibiotics that will block virus growth without killing the infected cell. However, in a few cases, compounds that specifically inhibit a viral process have been identified. These compounds are called *antivirals,* and they hold the key for future treatment of viral infections. As we shall see, an antiviral that inhibits HIV infection to some degree and slows down the progress of AIDS is *azidothymidine* (zidovudine), or *AZT.* At the present time, the basic treatment for a virus infection is to manage the symptoms and wait for the infection to run its course. Management of symptoms can include treatment to reduce fevers (for instance, aspirin), classical antibiotics (to prevent secondary infections by bacteria in a weakened individual), and bed rest.

Since treatment of virus infections is difficult, the best approach to managing viral disease is to prevent the initial infection. One powerful method is public health and sanitation methods to intervene in the epidemiological cycle of the virus, as described in Chapter 2. Another important approach is the use of viral *vaccines,* as described in Chapter 3. If immunity to a virus can be induced by the vaccine before a person encounters the virus, then it will not be able to establish a foothold. Some of the best-known virus vaccines are the smallpox vaccine developed by Edward Jenner (the first vaccine), the rabies vaccine developed by Louis Pasteur, and the polio vaccines developed by Jonas Salk and Albert Sabin.

THE LIFE CYCLE OF A RETROVIRUS

Human immunodeficiency virus belongs to a class of viruses called *retroviruses.* Let's examine the life cycle of a typical retrovirus.

The structure of a retrovirus is shown in Figure 4–4. The genetic information of a retrovirus is *RNA.* This RNA is covered with a viral *protein coat;* together, the viral RNA and protein coat make up a *core particle.* The core particle also contains several virus-specified enzymes. The core particle is surrounded by a viral *envelope,* which contains membrane lipids and viral envelope protein.

All retroviruses have three genes (see Figure 4–4). These genes code for:

1. *Coat proteins that make up the inner virus (core) particle.* The virus gene that specifies these proteins is called the *gag gene.* For HIV, there are three *gag proteins,* p17 (or MA), p24 (or CA), and p10 (or NC).

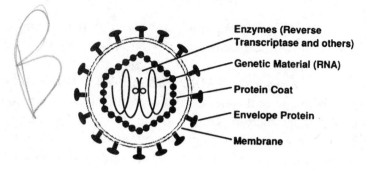

The RNA Genetic Material

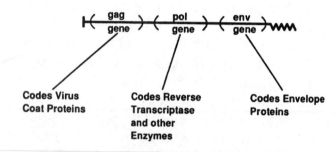

Figure 4–4

The structure of a retrovirus and its RNA genetic material.

2. *The enzyme reverse transcriptase, as well as some other enzymes used in virus replication.* The gene that codes these enzymes is the *pol* gene. The other viral enzymes specified by the *pol* gene are *protease* and *integrase*. **Protease** is involved in maturation of viral proteins as the virus particles bud from the cell, and integrase is responsible for integration of the viral DNA into the cell's chromosomal DNA.

3. *The proteins of the viral envelope.* The gene that codes for these proteins is the *env* gene. A protein coded by the *env* gene is responsible for binding the virus to the cell receptor. For HIV, there are two *env* proteins, gp120 and gp41.

It is important to discuss the *central dogma for genetic information flow* in cells. The central dogma states that genetic information flows in this direction:

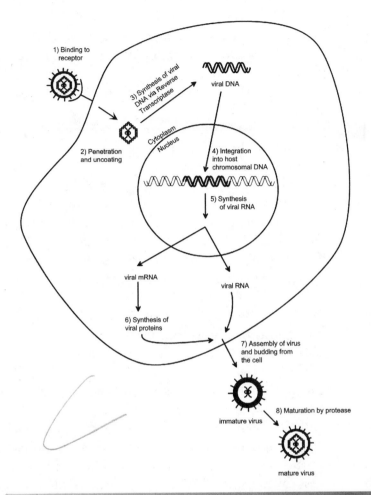

1) Binding to receptor

3) Synthesis of viral DNA via Reverse Transcriptase

viral DNA

2) Penetration and uncoating

Cytoplasm
Nucleus

4) Integration into host chromosomal DNA

5) Synthesis of viral RNA

viral mRNA

viral RNA

6) Synthesis of viral proteins

7) Assembly of virus and budding from the cell

immature virus

8) Maturation by protease

mature virus

Figure 4–5

The life cycle of a retrovirus.

$$DNA \rightarrow RNA \rightarrow Protein$$

That is, the genetic information is carried in *DNA* as a sequence of nucleotide bases (see Figure 3–9). In higher organisms, the DNA is organized into chromosomes that are located in the *nucleus* of the cell. When a gene is expressed, the information from the DNA base sequence is copied or transferred (transcribed) to a related molecule called *RNA* using the DNA molecule as a pattern. The RNA (which is called *messenger RNA* or *mRNA*) then moves from the cell nucleus to the *cytoplasm*. Once in the cytoplasm, the messenger RNA is used as a blueprint for the formation of *proteins* (translation). The proteins then carry out most of the important functions for the cell.

The life cycle of a retrovirus is shown in Figure 4–5. The retrovirus first binds to the surface of an uninfected cell by recognizing a cell receptor. After binding, the virus particle is brought into the cytoplasm of the cell. During this process, the viral envelope is removed, leaving the core particle. Once this happens, a unique virus-specified enzyme called *reverse transcriptase* is activated. This enzyme reads the viral RNA and makes *viral DNA*. The host cell lacks such an enzyme. The viral DNA then moves to the nucleus of the cell, where it is incorporated (or *integrated*) into the host cell's DNA in the chromosomes. Once this viral DNA is integrated into the chromosome, it resembles any other cell gene. As a result, the normal cell machinery reads the integrated viral DNA to make more copies of viral RNA. This viral RNA is then used for two purposes: (1) Some of the viral RNA moves to the cytoplasm and functions as *viral messenger RNA* to program the formation of *viral proteins,* and (2) the rest of the viral RNA becomes *genetic material* for new virus particles by moving to the cytoplasm and combining with viral proteins. These virus particles are formed at the cell surface and leave the cell by a process called *budding*. When virus particles initially bud from the cell, they are immature. This is because the viral proteins have not assumed their final form. The viral enzyme protease is responsible for conversion of immature virus particles into mature ones.

The retrovirus life cycle has several important characteristics. First, most retroviruses do not kill the cells they infect. Second, because viruses integrate their DNA into host chromosomes, they can establish a stable carrier state within the infected cell. As a result, once cells are infected with most retroviruses, they continually produce virus without dying. For some retroviruses, a latent state may also be established in which the retroviral DNA is integrated into the host chromosomes, but it does not program formation of new virus particles. However, at a later time (sometimes years later), the latent viral DNA may become activated by some means, and virus will be produced. This latency process is probably important in AIDS.

The viral enzyme *reverse transcriptase* carries out an unusual process in converting the viral RNA genetic information into DNA. This is the *reverse* of genetic information flow according to the central dogma of molecular biology, and this is the reason the enzyme is called reverse transcriptase. This is also where retro-viruses get their name—*retro* is from the Latin word for reverse.

THE AIDS VIRUS: HIV

The virus that causes AIDS is human immunodeficiency virus (HIV) (Figure 4–6). Other names that have been used previously for HIV include HTLV-III, LAV, and ARV. HIV belongs to a sub-group of retroviruses called *lentiviruses* (meaning *slow viruses,* since they often cause disease extremely slowly); other lentiviruses have been found in such diverse species as cats, sheep, goats, horses, and monkeys. The virus responsible for the great majority of AIDS cases in the United States, Europe, and Africa is called HIV-1. A second virus related to HIV-1 has been isolated in Africa: HIV-2 (see Chapters 4 and 6). HIV-2 also appears to cause AIDS. In this book, we will refer to the AIDS virus simply as HIV, and this will almost always mean HIV-1.

Features of HIV

Several features about the structure and replication of HIV are important (Figure 4–7a):

The Nature of the HIV Receptor
The cell receptor that HIV binds to is the *CD4 surface protein.* As described in Chapter 3, p. 25, CD4 protein is present on T_{helper} lymphocytes. In fact, this is the predominant cell type that has CD4 protein. In addition, some macrophages also have CD4 protein. Most other cells in the body do *not* contain CD4 protein. As a result, *the main cells that HIV can infect are T_{helper} lymphocytes and macrophages.* CD4 protein is also present on cells called dendritic cells, so they can also be infected with HIV. The HIV enve-

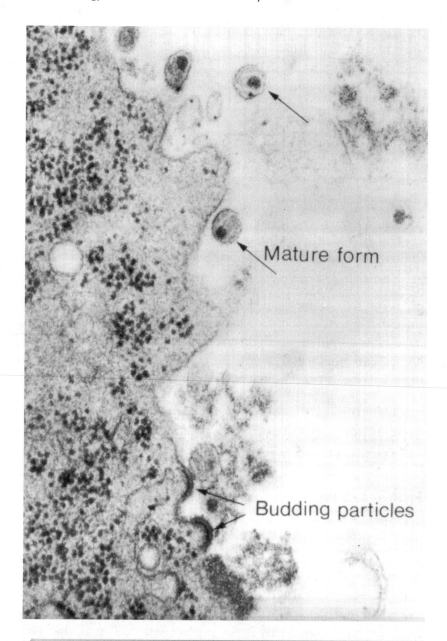

Mature form

Budding particles

Figure 4–6

An electron microscope picture of an HIV-infected cell. The cyto-plasm of the cell is on the left, and the exterior of the cell is on the right. Budding HIV particles are indicated, as well as mature virus particles released from the cell. The cores of mature HIV particles have a conical shape. *(Courtesy of the Centers for Disease Control)*

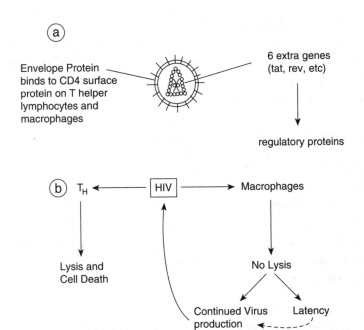

Envelope Protein binds to CD4 surface protein on T helper lymphocytes and macrophages

6 extra genes (tat, rev, etc)

regulatory proteins

(b) T_H ← HIV → Macrophages

Lysis and Cell Death

No Lysis

Continued Virus production   Latency

(Reactivation)

Figure 4–7

Unusual features of HIV.

lope protein responsible for virus binding to CD4 protein is called gp120.

Additional Genes

As all retroviruses do, HIV contains the three genes for coat proteins, reverse transcriptase, and envelope proteins. In addition, HIV contains genes that specify six additional proteins. These are regulatory proteins that give HIV finer levels of control and a more versatile life cycle. Two of the best-known of these genes are *tat*, which is an up-regulator or amplifier of viral gene expression in the infected cell, and *rev*, which shifts the balance from production of viral regulatory proteins to proteins that make up virus particles.

The other HIV genes specify proteins called *nef, vpu, vif,* and *vpr.* Some facilitate the infection process in different ways. Others may be important in allowing the virus to establish a latent or inactive state in some infected cells, followed by reactivation at later times.

Killing of T$_{helper}$ Lymphocytes

In contrast to most retroviral infections, *infection of T$_{helper}$ lymphocytes with HIV results in cell death* (Figure 4–7b). Considering the pivotal role that T$_{helper}$ lymphocytes play in both humoral and cell-mediated immunity (see Chapter 3, p. 45), it is possible to understand how infection with HIV can ultimately lead to collapse of the immune system.

Nonlytic Infection of Macrophages

When HIV infects macrophages, it follows a course that is typical of other retroviruses, in that the infected macrophages are not killed (see Figure 4–7b). In most cases, the macrophages continue to produce HIV virus particles, while other macrophages establish a latent state of HIV infection. These infected macrophages are an important reservoir of infection in an HIV-infected individual.

Co-receptors for HIV

As described above, when HIV infects a cell, it must bind to the CD4 protein. However, binding to the CD4 protein alone will not result in entry of the HIV virus particle into a cell. The cell must have an additional protein on its cell surface for virus entry to take place—a co-receptor. As shown in Figure 4–8, a cell must express both CD4 protein and a co-receptor in order to be infected. The *co-receptors for HIV* turn out to be proteins that normally bind particular cell growth factors. As discussed in Chapter 3, specific growth factors are required for the growth of different blood cells (e.g. IL-2 for T$_{helper}$ lymphocytes); these growth factors signal for cell growth by binding to receptor proteins on the cell surface. The HIV co-receptor on T$_{helper}$ lymphocytes is a growth factor receptor called *CXCR4*, and the co-receptor on macrophages is a receptor called *CCR5*.

The Effects of HIV Infection in Individuals

Let's now consider the results of HIV infection at the level of infected people. The routes of HIV infection are covered in Chapters 6 and 7, so here we will start at the time a person becomes infected. There is a detailed description of AIDS as a clinical disease in Chapter 5, but an overview is useful at this point.

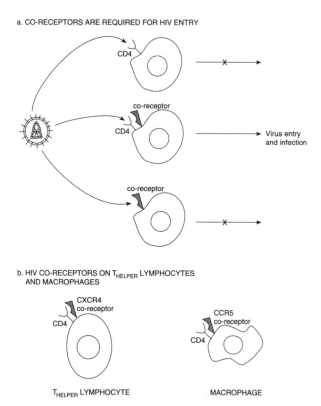

a. CO-RECEPTORS ARE REQUIRED FOR HIV ENTRY

b. HIV CO-RECEPTORS ON T$_{HELPER}$ LYMPHOCYTES AND MACROPHAGES

Figure 4–8

Co-receptors for HIV infection. In addition to the CD4 protein, cells must also have a co-receptor for HIV infection. The co-receptor on T$_{helper}$ lymphocytes is the CXCR4, and the co-receptor on macrophages is CCR5.

The progression of events after HIV infection is shown in Figure 4–9. After HIV infection, there is often (but not always) an acute infection syndrome typified by a mild flu-like illness or swollen glands, which goes away after a few weeks. Many HIV-infected people do not associate the symptoms of the acute infection syndrome with HIV infection. Most individuals then remain free of any clinical symptoms for variable lengths of time, typically many years. Individuals who are HIV infected but who do not show any signs of disease are referred to as *asymptomatic*. It is generally difficult to detect infectious HIV virus in the blood of infected asymptomatic individuals. Indeed, even as individuals de-

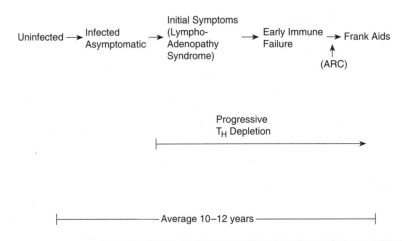

Figure 4–9

Consequences of HIV infection in the absence of antiviral therapy.

velop clinical symptoms, they generally have rather low levels of infectious HIV in the blood. In the beginning, one of the puzzles about HIV was how it could cause such devastating disease with such apparently low levels of circulating virus. This topic is discussed further in Chapter 5. During the asymptomatic period, individuals generally produce *antibodies* to HIV. Unfortunately, these antibodies are not sufficient to prevent continued HIV infection as the disease progresses. However, they provide a useful diagnosis for HIV infection, as we shall see later.

As time passes, many HIV-infected individuals begin to experience symptoms of HIV infection. Some initial symptoms include persistent enlarged lymph glands (*lymphoadenopathy syndrome* or *LAS*) and fevers or night sweats. As the disease worsens, a continuum of progressively more serious conditions develops as the immune system weakens, ultimately resulting in full-blown AIDS. During the early periods of the AIDS epidemic, doctors also used a classification called *ARC* or *AIDS-related complex*. Individuals were classified as having ARC if they showed fewer of the characteristic opportunistic infections or cancers (see below) than patients with full-blown AIDS. The term *ARC* is not used today. The progression from asymptomatic infection to AIDS is accompanied by a progressive depletion of

T_{helper} lymphocytes by HIV infection. Ultimately, there is a profound lack of T_{helper} lymphocytes, which results in the failure of both humoral and cell-mediated immunity. In individuals with normal immune systems, the T_{helper} counts are typically over 1,000 per cubic millimeter of blood, while in patients with full-blown AIDS, these may be well under 100 per cubic millimeter.

The clinical manifestations of AIDS are covered in detail in Chapter 5. They are summarized briefly here:

Opportunistic infections: These are infections by microorganisms that normally do not cause problems in healthy individuals. However, in individuals with weakened immune systems, these microorganisms can take hold and cause devastating infections. One frequent opportunistic infection is *Pneumocystis carinii* (*PCP pneumonia*), caused by a fungus microbe.

Cancers: Cell-mediated immunity also plays an important role in defense against development of cancers (immune surveillance; see Chapter 3, p. 42). HIV-infected individuals develop several cancers with very high frequency. One example of an AIDS-related cancer is *Kaposi's sarcoma.*

Weight loss: Many AIDS patients suffer from profound weight loss or wasting. The mechanism for this is not yet understood.

Mental impairment: HIV can also establish infection in the nervous system. This can result in muscle spasms or tics. More serious is infection of the central nervous system, which can result in *AIDS-related dementia,* in which individuals lose the ability to reason.

Individual AIDS patients may suffer from one or more of these manifestations. Indeed, they may experience recurrent bouts with different opportunistic infections or cancers.

Since the major problem in AIDS is a loss of T_{helper} lymphocyte function, monitoring of the numbers of T_{helper} lymphocytes is important in HIV-infected individuals. Doctors can perform a test for these cells, and the results are reported in terms of T_{helper} (or T4 or CD4) lymphocyte numbers. Early in the epidemic, the tests were frequently reported as the ratio of T_{helper} to T_{killer} lymphocytes in the blood (also T4/T8 or helper-to-suppressor ratios). An inversion of the normal T_{helper}/T_{killer} lymphocyte ratio is often an early sign of HIV infection.

The likelihood that an HIV-infected individual will develop full-blown AIDS is discussed in more detail in Chapter 6. Current estimates are that without treatment, more than 90 percent of HIV-infected individuals will develop AIDS with an average time to disease of ten to twelve years.

One of the early enigmas of HIV infection and AIDS was that, until the disease has progressed quite far, very little infectious HIV is apparent in the blood of an infected individual. This fact even led some people to question whether HIV is the cause of AIDS, although the epidemiological and clinical results make it very clear that this is the case. However, recent studies with advanced techniques have shown that there is extensive infection of T-lymphocytes in lymph nodes, although the infected cells and the infectious virus are not released into the bloodstream until late in the disease.

The HIV Antibody Test

Within a year of the isolation of HIV as the causative agent of AIDS, a test was developed that determines if an individual has been exposed to HIV. The procedure is to test whether an individual has antibodies to HIV virus proteins. These antibodies appear in those who have been previously infected with HIV and have made antibodies against the virus (see Chapter 3, pp. 37–40).

The most common HIV antibody test is called an *ELISA* test, shown in Figure 4–10. In an ELISA assay, virus protein is first attached to a small laboratory dish. A serum sample is prepared from the blood of the individual to be tested, and it is placed in the dish containing bound HIV viral proteins. If HIV-specific antibodies are present in the serum, they will become tightly bound to the dish by way of the HIV proteins. The serum is then removed, and the dish is washed. During this procedure, only antibodies specific for HIV will be retained. The dish is then reacted with a stain that will detect *any* human antibodies. Thus, dishes that were exposed to serum containing HIV-specific antibodies will be stained, but dishes from antibody-negative serum

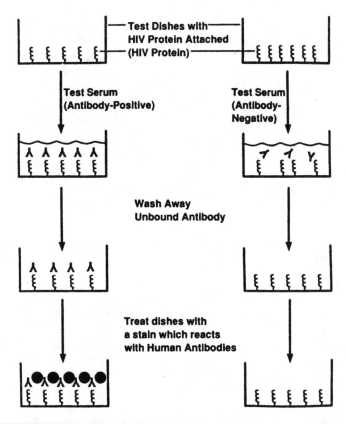

Figure 4–10

The ELISA test for HIV antibody.

samples will be unstained. This procedure has been automated, so that many blood samples can be tested at once (Figure 4–11). The current ELISA tests are better than 99.9 percent accurate. That is, fewer than 0.1 percent of HIV-negative individuals incorrectly score as positive by the ELISA test. Likewise, fewer than 0.1 percent of HIV antibody-positive serum samples are missed by the test.

Potential Problems with the HIV Antibody Test

Although this test has been extremely important in furthering our knowledge of how the virus spreads and causes disease and in identifying HIV-infected people, it has several potential problems.

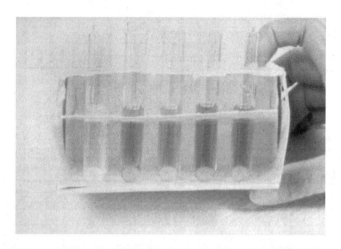

Figure 4–11

A modified ELISA test is shown. In this case, the virus proteins are attached to small beads that can float in solution, instead of on the bottom of the dish. The tube on the left shows a test of a blood sample that does not have HIV-specific antibodies. The four tubes on the right show test of HIV antibody-positive blood samples. The color in the tubes on the right indicates the presence of HIV antibodies. *(Courtesy of Abbot Laboratories, Diagnostic Division)*

False Positives

These are individuals who are not HIV-infected but who test antibody-positive in the ELISA assay. Clearly, this can be an extremely frightening experience. With current ELISA assays, the frequency of false positives is less than 1 in 1,000 (0.1 percent) uninfected individuals. False positives are a particular problem if populations with low frequencies of HIV infection are tested. In these cases, a high proportion of the individuals who score positive could be false positives. This is one of the arguments (besides cost) against routine HIV antibody screening of the general U.S. population, where current prevalences of infection are less than 1 percent—many of the individuals identified as antibody positive in such a mass screening could actually be false positives.

Because of the significant false positive rate for the ELISA test, a second, more specific test for HIV antibodies is also used:

the *Western blot* test. This technique has a lower incidence of false positives than the ELISA assay. In practice, serum samples that score antibody positive by the ELISA test are generally retested by the Western blot procedure. Serum samples are considered positive if they are found to contain HIV-specific antibodies by both tests. New and improved tests (more sensitive and/or more accurate) for HIV infection are currently undergoing development (see below).

False Negatives

A more important problem is individuals who are infected with HIV but who do not score positive in the HIV antibody test. Such individuals fall into two categories:

1. *Recently infected individuals.* As was discussed in Chapter 3, the immune system has a lag period between initial exposure to an antigen and the production of antibodies. In the case of HIV infection, this lag can range up to six months or longer. Thus, individuals who have been recently infected with HIV will not score positive in the antibody test.

2. *Infected individuals who never mount an immune response.* Since the immune response varies from person to person, a few infected individuals do not produce antibodies to HIV. There are rare but documented cases of individuals who remain antibody negative but spread HIV infection to their sexual partners.

The HIV antibody test measures whether an individual has circulating antibodies to HIV. However, strictly speaking, the test does *not* indicate if an antibody-positive individual still harbors infectious virus. Some individuals who are exposed to HIV might have raised a successful immune response and completely eliminated the infection. However, by and large, most HIV-antibody positive individuals turn out to be still infected.

Testing for the Level of Circulating HIV

While the HIV antibody test is routinely used to identify individuals who have been exposed to HIV, other tests for viral infection are used as well. In particular, it is advantageous to know the amount of circulating virus particles in an infected individual, since the levels of virus are generally low, but they frequently rise when full-blown AIDS develops. The most common test for virus particles is to measure the level of the major HIV core protein (p24 protein) in the blood. Because this test detects p24 protein by use of an antibody against it, it is often referred to as a test for p24 antigen.

More sensitive tests for HIV infection have been developed. These are based on a technique called *polymerase chain reaction* or *PCR*, which tests for HIV DNA in infected cells or for HIV RNA in virus particles. One application of the PCR tests has been to detect infected cells in HIV-infected individuals. The sensitivity of the PCR test is important because in an HIV-infected individual, most cells are not infected—even among CD4-positive T_h lymphocytes and monocytes/macrophages. The PCR test can detect as few as one HIV-infected cell among a million uninfected ones.

More recently, another version of the PCR test has been developed that detects HIV RNA in virus particles. This test is used to detect the very low levels of virus in the blood of asymptomatic individuals. As is discussed in Chapter 5, p. 84, the level of HIV RNA in the blood of infected people (sometimes called the *viral RNA load*) has become an important measure for assessing progression of disease and the effectiveness of antiviral therapies in an infected person.

How Does HIV Evade the Immune System?

One of the paradoxes about HIV infection is that most infected individuals contain HIV antibodies, but the disease eventually occurs in most cases, even in the presence of these antibodies. This means that HIV antibodies are unable to prevent onset of AIDS. This may be due to several factors. First, the levels of antibodies raised might be insufficient to block the spread of infectious virus. In addition, antibodies can be produced against different parts of the virus. Only some of these antibodies (*neutralizing antibodies*) can inactivate virus and prevent infection. Finally, several unique features of HIV infection provide the virus with ways to evade the immune system.

High Mutation Rates
The HIV envelope proteins are on the outside of the virus particle, and they are important in attaching the virus to the cell receptor.

As such, they are the most important targets for neutralizing antibodies. HIV has an unusually high mutation rate, estimated as one DNA base mutation each time an HIV DNA molecule is made by reverse transcriptase. The consequence of this process is that mutations in the HIV *env* gene occur very frequently, so that the exact amino acid sequence of the envelope proteins changes quite rapidly during successive cycles of infection. Equivalent mutations in the *gag* and *pol* genes generally are not compatible with virus survival. Changes in the makeup of HIV envelope proteins have even been observed over time within the same person. Thus, even though an infected individual may raise neutralizing antibodies to the initial infecting virus, those antibodies may not be able to neutralize subsequent viruses with mutated envelope proteins. Thus, HIV can keep one step ahead of the immune system and continue infection.

Latent States

HIV can establish *latent states* in some cells. In these cells, the viral DNA is maintained, but virus proteins are not expressed. As a result, these latently infected cells will not be recognized or attacked by the immune system but will remain as reservoirs for infectious virus. At later times, the virus may be activated from these cells. Macrophages are probably the major cells that carry latent HIV, since initial HIV infection does not kill them. In addition, T_{helper} cells latently infected with HIV may also exist, although in fewer numbers than latently infected macrophages.

Reactivation of latent HIV from carrier cells may also be important in AIDS progression. Infection of cells carrying latent HIV with certain other viruses, such as herpes simplex or cytomegalovirus, may reactivate the HIV. In addition, other stimuli to the immune system (such as infection with other microorganisms) can result in production of factors that reactivate HIV. These secondary infections may be important cofactors in AIDS progression.

Cell-to-Cell Spread

HIV can carry out infection by *cell-to-cell spread*. That is, if an HIV-infected cell comes into contact with an uninfected cell, the virus may pass to the uninfected cell directly. Neutralizing antibodies are unable to prevent this process, since they can attack virus only when it is outside cells.

These properties of HIV also pose another problem. Vaccines are our front line of defense against most virus infections, as described earlier in this chapter. However, the ability of HIV to evade the immune system means that it will much more difficult to design an effective anti-HIV vaccine.

AZIDOTHYMIDINE (AZT), AN EFFECTIVE THERAPEUTIC AGENT IN AIDS

The first successful drug against HIV infection and AIDS was azidothymidine (or zidovudine, or AZT, or Retrovir). The effectiveness and use of AZT are described in more detail in Chapters 5 and 6. However, let's consider its mode of action here.

Azidothymidine is very similar in chemical structure to thymidine, one of the building blocks of DNA. However, when AZT is incorporated in place of thymidine during the DNA assembly process, its structure aborts further DNA assembly. This inactivates any growing DNA molecule that has incorporated AZT. During HIV infection, if AZT is present, HIV reverse transcriptase will readily incorporate it into the viral DNA. This will inactivate the viral DNA. It is important that the enzymes responsible for making the chromosomal DNA of the cell (cellular DNA polymerases) do *not* efficiently incorporate AZT into DNA. As a result, the cell can continue to grow and make its genetic material, but HIV cannot replicate efficiently if AZT is present. Thus, AZT is a *selective poison* for HIV. It exploits an "Achilles heel" of the virus—reverse transcriptase. This enzyme plays no role in the uninfected cell, but it is vital to the virus. An agent that affects this enzyme will have no effect on the uninfected cell but will inhibit virus infection. This is shown in Figure 4–12.

Limitations of AZT

Although AZT is an effective drug in AIDS treatment, it has some limitations:

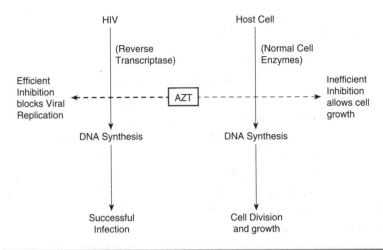

Figure 4–12

The action of AZT.

Toxic side effects. Normal cellular DNA polymerases do not efficiently incorporate AZT into DNA in comparison to HIV reverse transcriptase—the basis for the drug's selectivity. However, cellular DNA polymerases do incorporate some AZT into cell DNA at low levels. During prolonged treatment, this can lead to death of normal cells. *Anemia* is a common side effect in individuals taking AZT; it results from killing of blood cells by the drug.

Inability to halt progression to AIDS. AZT treatment improves the clinical condition of individuals with full-blown AIDS, but it is not a cure (see Chapter 5, p. 103). The inability of AZT to halt progression to AIDS is related to the fact that the virus can mutate in the individual. Indeed, AZT-resistant HIV develops in individuals who have been taking AZT.

Development of AZT-resistant variants. As described above, HIV has a high mutation rate. Normally, few mutations in the *pol* gene appear because they decrease the virus's growth rate if they occur. However, under the selective pressure of AZT, AZT-resistant variants of HIV appear that have mutated reverse transcriptase. This mutated enzyme does not incorporate AZT as efficiently, making the virus less sensitive to the drug. AZT-resistant HIV variants have been detected in AIDS patients who are taking AZT, and these variants contribute to the inability of AZT to prevent the effects of HIV indefinitely.

Despite its limitations, the effectiveness of AZT in treating AIDS patients has a very important implication. Even in individuals who are already infected, *prevention of continued HIV infection improves the clinical status.* Thus, other drugs that selectively inhibit HIV reverse transcriptase will be useful therapeutic agents. Moreover, the other HIV proteins are all potential "Achilles heels" for the virus as well. Agents that interfere with the action of any of these proteins may also be useful therapeutic agents. AIDS researchers are devoting a great deal of effort to developing new anti-HIV drugs.

Following initial success of AZT in inhibiting HIV replication and improving the clinical condition of AIDS patients, several other drugs that work by the same general mechanism have been developed and approved for use. These include *dideoxycytidine (ddC), dideoxyinosine (ddI), 3TC (lamivudine)* and *D4T (stavudine).* The active forms of these drugs are preferentially incorporated into viral DNA by HIV reverse transcriptase, and they all prevent further DNA synthesis. As a class, these drugs (including AZT) are referred to as *nucleoside analogs.* Different nucleoside analogs are incorporated into HIV DNA in place of different DNA bases; for instance ddC is incorporated into HIV DNA in place of the base cytosine (or C).

PROTEASE INHIBITORS, ANOTHER CLASS OF THERAPEUTIC AGENTS AGAINST HIV

In 1996, a new class of anti-HIV drugs completed development and reached the market: *protease inhibitors.* These drugs are targeted on the viral enzyme protease. Earlier in this chapter (pp. 57–61), we learned that the protease is important for the conversion of immature virus particles to mature ones (see Figure 4–5). In fact, if this maturation does not take place, the immature HIV particles are not infectious. Thus, drugs that inhibit the protease enzyme will inhibit production of infectious HIV.

A more detailed view of the role of protease in viral maturation is shown in Figure 4–13. When the viral proteins specified by

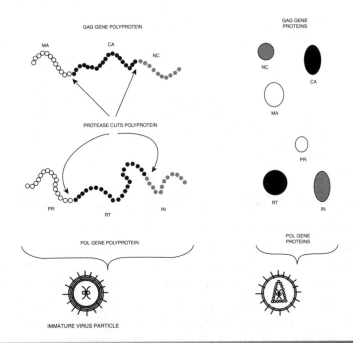

GAG GENE POLYPROTEIN

GAG GENE
PROTEINS

PROTEASE CUTS POLYPROTEIN

POL GENE POLYPROTEIN

POL GENE
PROTEINS

IMMATURE VIRUS PARTICLE

Figure 4–13

Maturation of HIV particles by protease. The role of protease in cutting the *gag* and *pol* gene polyproteins to give the proteins of the mature HIV particle is shown. The abbreviations for the viral proteins are: MA (matrix) = p17; CA (caspid) = p24; NC (nucleocaspid) = p10; PR = protease; RT = reverse transcriptase; IN = integrase. Note that the shape of the core in the mature HIV particle is conical.

the *gag* gene are initially made in the infected cell, they are in the form of one long chain of amino acids (see also Figure 3–7). That is, the amino acids for one *gag* protein are attached to the next gag protein in one long string, referred to as a *polyprotein*. The same is true of the viral proteins specified by the *pol* gene. In fact, when the virus particles initially form, it is the viral polyproteins that combine with viral RNA to make the immature virus particles that bud from the infected cell. The viral protease liberates the individual *gag* and *pol* gene proteins from the polyproteins by cutting between specific amino acids.

The protease inhibitors work by binding to the HIV protease enzyme and directly inhibiting its function. This differs from the way in which nucleoside analogs such as AZT inhibit HIV replication. Nucleoside analogs do not actually inhibit reverse transcriptase, but they take advantage of the fact that reverse transcriptase will preferentially incorporate them into growing HIV DNA and inactivate it. Four protease inhibitors have been approved for treatment of HIV-infected individuals. They have made a significant improvement in treatment and are discussed in greater detail in Chapter 5.

WHERE DID HIV COME FROM?

Molecular biologists have examined the genetic structure of HIV (actually HIV-1 and HIV-2) in great detail and compared it to the structure of other retroviruses of the lentivirus subclass. From these studies, it is clear that HIV has a common origin with other lentiviruses, and they evolved from a common ancestral retrovirus over millions of years. In particular, HIV-1 and HIV-2 represent recent infections in humans of lentiviruses native to African primates (*simian immunodeficiency virus, or SIVs*). HIV-1 came from infection in humans of an SIV from chimpanzees, and HIV-2 came from an SIV of sooty mangabeys. Epidemiological studies tell us that fifteen to twenty years ago, HIV-1 spread into high-density populations in Africa and the Western world, leading to the AIDS epidemic. Recent changes in human social behavior, such as the sexual revolution, may have also contributed to the spread of HIV infection.

Numerous apocryphal stories as to the origin of HIV have circulated since the beginning of the AIDS epidemic. These include: HIV was the result of germ warfare research by the CIA; HIV was a laboratory accident involving recombinant DNA; HIV resulted from a plot between Israel and South Africa; HIV resulted from sexual relations between humans and sheep; and HIV resulted from sexual relations between humans and monkeys. *None of these are true.*

Chapter 5
Clinical Manifestations of AIDS

 **A. EXPOSURE, INFECTION, AND DISEASE**

   i. Exposure Versus Infection

   ii. Infection Versus Disease

 **B. PRIMARY INFECTION AND THE ASYMPTOMATIC PERIOD**

   i. Mononucleosis-like Illness

   ii. Brain Infection (Encephalopathy)

   iii. The Asymptomatic Period

 **C. INITIAL DISEASE SYMPTOMS**

   i. Wasting Syndrome

   ii. Lymphadenopathy Syndrome

   iii. Neurological Disease

 **D. DAMAGE TO THE IMMUNE SYSTEM AND FULL-BLOWN AIDS**

   i. Early Immune Failure

   ii. Full-blown AIDS

      a. Fungal Infections

In Chapters 3 and 4, we learned about AIDS at the cellular and subcellular levels. In particular, cells of the immune system were discussed, and the effects of HIV infection on those cells were presented. With that background, we can now consider the effects of HIV in terms of a whole person—the actual symptoms that infected individuals experience. A brief overview of AIDS at the organismal level is included in Chapter 4, and in this chapter, a detailed description of the clinical manifestations of AIDS is presented. The physical manifestations of the disease are of great importance to AIDS patients and their health-care providers, but it is important to remember the human side of the disease as well. AIDS is often a fatal disease. For persons to learn that they are infected with HIV evokes tremendous emotional stress. Counselors are trained to help patients deal with this psychologically difficult situation. In this chapter, we simply present the biological or clinical aspects of AIDS.

EXPOSURE, INFECTION, AND DISEASE

In terms of AIDS and HIV at the organismal level, it is important to consider interaction of the virus with a susceptible individual. Three important concepts in the interaction are *exposure, infection,* and *disease.*

Exposure Versus Infection

When an HIV-infected individual encounters an uninfected person, this does not always result in transmission of HIV to the uninfected person. Indeed, even if exposure occurs by one of the three routes known to transmit the virus (blood, birth, and sex), only a fraction of exposed people will be infected. The relative risk factors affecting the efficiency of HIV transmission are discussed in Chapters 6 and 7. As we shall see, different kinds of exposure between infected and uninfected individuals have different probabilities of leading to infection.

As introduced in Chapter 4, most individuals who are exposed to HIV and become infected do not realize they are infected right away. It is generally not possible to distinguish infected and uninfected people simply on the basis of their physical well-being. The HIV antibody test is invaluable in identifying individuals infected with HIV (see Chapter 4, p. 68). Generally, an infected person will begin to produce antibodies against HIV *(seroconvert)* two to three months after infection, although the time for seroconversion is variable and can last as long as a year or more. In practical terms, someone who was exposed to HIV is generally considered to be uninfected if he or she is seronegative for HIV antibodies six months after the last exposure to HIV and remains seronegative for another six months during which no other potential exposures occur.

Infection Versus Disease

Even among individuals who become infected with a virus, not necessarily everybody will develop physical symptoms. With many viruses, most of the infected individuals actually never develop physical signs of illness. Unfortunately, most people infected with HIV ultimately develop some disease symptoms (see Chapter 6).

The disease symptoms that result from virus infection are caused by destruction or damage of cells and tissues in the infected person. In some cases, the damage may result from direct killing of cells by the infecting virus. In other cases, the physical symptoms may result from indirect effects of the virus. In the case of AIDS, most of the physical symptoms are the indirect results of damage to the immune system by HIV (see Chapters 3 and 4).

Many virus infections can cause a variety of physical symptoms. Other factors can influence the exact nature of the symptoms in a particular individual, including age, sex, genetic makeup, nutrition, environmental factors, and encounters with other infectious agents. As we shall see, this is particularly true for AIDS, in which the symptoms result from indirect immunological damage.

A schematic diagram of the different clinical stages of HIV infection is shown in Figure 5–1. In time sequence, the stages can be grouped into three categories: (1) *initial infection and the asymptomatic period,* (2) *initial symptoms,* and (3) *immunological damage* (early signs through full-blown AIDS).

PRIMARY INFECTION AND THE ASYMPTOMATIC PERIOD

Some people who become infected with HIV never experience any symptoms at the time of initial infection. On the other hand, other HIV-infected people do develop some relatively mild disease symptoms right after infection (before seroconversion). These are referred to as *acute symptoms,* and they generally last only a few days and then disappear. Two types of acute symptoms can occur.

Initial Infection

) Transient early (acute) symptoms

Asymptomatic

Initial Symptoms

1. Lymphadenopathy

2. Wasting syndrome / Fever / Night sweats

3. Neurological disease

Early immune failure

1. Shingles (VZV)

2. Thrush (Candida)

3. Hairy Leukoplakia (EBV)

Frank AIDS (Opportunistic infection)

1. Pneumonia (Pneumocystis)

2. Kaposi's sarcoma

3. Other protozoan infections

4. Systemic Fungal infection

5. Bacterial infection (TB like)

6. Viral infection (CMV)

7. Other cancer (lymphoma)

Figure 5–1

The progression of symptoms in AIDS. (These symptoms may be additive.)

Mononucleosis-like Illness

The most common early illness seen with HIV infection resembles another viral disease, mononucleosis. Mononucleosis is not exclusive to a particular virus in that other viral infections can cause these symptoms as well. The most prominent symptoms are swollen lymph glands. In the case of HIV infection, this includes lymph glands throughout the body—called generalized *lymphadenopathy*. In addition, there may also be a sore throat, a fever, and a skin rash. Because these symptoms also result from infection by other viruses, it is not possible to diagnose an HIV infection solely based on the appearance of these symptoms.

Brain Infection (Encephalopathy)

HIV infection of the brain can occur at this early time and lead to brain swelling or inflammation, particularly of the brain lining or meninges. In medical terms, this is called *encephalopathy*. Macrophage cells in the brain appear to be prominent sites for virus replication. The brain inflammation may result from the influx of immune system cells to fight the infection or the release from infected cells of highly active molecules that can affect other brain cells. The brain inflammation causes symptoms of headache and fever. Brain function can be impaired to various degrees. Often the person will have difficulty concentrating, remembering, or solving problems. Some personality changes may also occur during the acute phase.

The Asymptomatic Period

During the acute phase of infection, significant levels of circulating infectious HIV are generally detectable in the blood. Following the acute phase, the levels of infectious virus in the blood decrease, often to undetectable levels. The infected person usually feels well but becomes *serpositive* for HIV. This is referred to as the period of *asymptomatic infection*. As mentioned earlier, the asymptomatic period may last as long as ten or more years or sometimes less than one year. We do not understand why there is such variability.

During the asymptomatic period, some type of balance is established between HIV infection and the immune system in the infected person. Ultimately, for most individuals, changes in the virus or the immune system allow the HIV infection to escape from control and lead to disease.

With the recent development of the sensitive PCR assays for HIV virus particles, it has become clear that although most asymptomatic HIV-infected people have very low or undetectable levels of infectious HIV in their blood, they *do* actually have low but measurable levels of circulating virus particles. Those particles may or may not be infectious. As described in Chapter 4, p. 71, the level of circulating HIV particles in the blood as measured by the PCR assay is referred to as the viral RNA load. Different asymptomatic individuals have different levels of viral RNA load in the blood that typically are relatively constant throughout the asymptomatic phase. Increases in the viral RNA loads occur as infected individuals progress towards AIDS. Asymptomatic HIV-infected people with high viral loads progress to clinical AIDS faster than individuals with low viral loads. As a result, viral load measurements have become important in treating and monitoring asymptomatic HIV-infected individuals. We will return to this later (see pp. 106–108).

INITIAL DISEASE SYMPTOMS

The initial disease that follows the asymptomatic period falls into three major classes. An infected person may have symptoms of more than one of these classes.

Wasting Syndrome

The two symptoms seen with this syndrome are a sudden and otherwise unexplained *loss in body weight* (more than 10 percent of total body weight) and *fevers*, usually at night, that cause *night sweats*. The weight loss is usually progressive, leading to wasting away of the infected person, and may be accompanied by diarrhea. This wasting syndrome is very reminiscent of the progressive loss of body weight by cancer patients. The fevers can involve dangerously high temperatures (106–107° Fahrenheit), which can result in brain damage. Normally, the body controls high internal temperatures by sweating. The night sweats result from the bodies of infected individuals lowering their temperatures by sweating.

Lymphadenopathy Syndrome

As described above, *lymphadenopathy* means swelling of the lymph glands. Lymphadenopathy sometimes is also an acute symptom of HIV infection, but in lymphadenopathy syndrome (*LAS*), the lymph gland enlargement is persistent. This condition as also called *persistent generalized lymphadenopathy* or *PGL*. In LAS, the lymph glands in the head and neck, the armpits, and the groin are usually swollen, although they generally are not painful. Some infected people experience both LAS and the wasting syndrome described above. In the past, lymphadenopathy was one of a group of symptoms that was associated with AIDS-related complex (ARC; see Chapter 4), a condition considered less serious than AIDS. However, the term *ARC* is not used nowadays, and lymphadenopathy actually can occur at various stages of the disease.

Neurological Disease

The HIV infection can spread to the brain and either damage the brain directly or lead to damage by other infectious agents. In addition, other parts of the nervous system can be damaged and cause different neurological symptoms. About one-third of all AIDS patients have some of the following neurological symptoms:

> *Dementia.* When the brain itself is damaged, mental functions are impaired. With HIV infection, this is usually a progressive situation. Initially, this may appear as simple forgetfulness about where things are. As the disease progresses, the loss of mental function can become more serious: The infected person may have difficulty reasoning and performing other mental tasks. Depression, social withdrawal, and personality changes are also common. Eventually, as the disease progresses, infected people may become demented and unable to care for themselves. For some AIDS

patients, this progression leads to the patient entering a coma followed by death, if other infections or cancers do not kill the patient first. Death usually occurs several months after the onset of dementia.

Spinal cord damage (myelopathy). Because the spinal cord transmits nerve impulses to the muscles of the body, damage to the spinal cord can result in weakness or paralysis of voluntary muscles. As a result, HIV infection can lead to spinal cord swelling (*myelopathy*) and paralysis or weakness of the limbs.

Peripheral nerve damage (neuropathy). Some people infected with HIV experience swelling (neuropathy) of the peripheral nerves. These nerves are involved in sensing pain. When they are damaged, they can cause burning or stinging sensations, usually in the hands or feet. In addition, numbness, especially in the feet, is frequent.

These initial symptoms of HIV infection are not mutually exclusive. Individual patients may experience a mixture of any of them.

DAMAGE TO THE IMMUNE SYSTEM AND FULL-BLOWN AIDS

As described in Chapter 4, the major problem in HIV infection is damage to the immune system. Two major consequences result from immunological damage: the occurrence of *opportunistic infections,* caused by infectious agents that are normally held in check by healthy immune systems, and the development of *cancers* that also result from failure of the immune system (see Chapter 3, pp. 42–44). In HIV-infected individuals, both opportunistic infections and cancers may develop (sometimes at the same time), but opportunistic infections are generally the more common cause of death.

As indicated in Chapter 4, the breakdown of the immune system in HIV-infected individuals is a continuous and gradual process. It generally begins with relatively minor opportunistic infections and usually progresses to severe and life-threatening disease—full-blown AIDS. After the isolation of HIV, an early medical definition for diagnosing AIDS was evidence of HIV infection (seropositivity) in conjunction with two or more serious opportunistic infections or cancers. This was initially used by epidemiologists and clinicians in staging and classifying the disease. However, we now know that AIDS represents the final and most severe symptoms of HIV infection, and it is not really distinct from other manifestations of HIV disease. In 1993, a new AIDS definition was added: evidence of HIV infection (seropositivity) and T_{helper} counts below 200 per cubic millimeter. In adults, full-blown AIDS almost never occurs before two years of infection.

Early Immune Failure

Previously, the term *ARC* was sometimes used to describe the relatively minor infections or the lesser manifestations of immune system failure. Following are some of the more common opportunistic infections that occur during early immune failure.

Candida. *Candida* is a genus of fungus, similar to baker's yeast, that can be found on the skin and mucosal surfaces (mouth, vagina) of most people. Normally, *Candida* growth is held in check by an ecological balance with other microorganisms and by the immune system. In AIDS patients, *Candida* often infects the mouth, causing a condition known as *candidiasis* or *thrush*. With thrush, the *Candida* will form white plaques in the mouth that feel furry to the patient (Figure 5–2). Antifungal drugs such as mycostatin are used to control these infections, although they are difficult to completely eliminate. HIV-infected people who develop candidiasis have a high probability of progressing to full-blown AIDS. Often, the infection can spread down the esophagus and cause a very painful burning sensation when the patient eats. This condition is known as *esophagitis*; patients with esophagitis are generally considered to have full-blown AIDS. Approximately 50 percent of AIDS patients will experience, at some time, a Candida infection.

In HIV-infected women, vaginal Candida infections are a very important symptom.

Shingles (varicella). *Shingles* or *varicella* is a painful rash condition that often occurs on the torso (Figure 5–3). It is

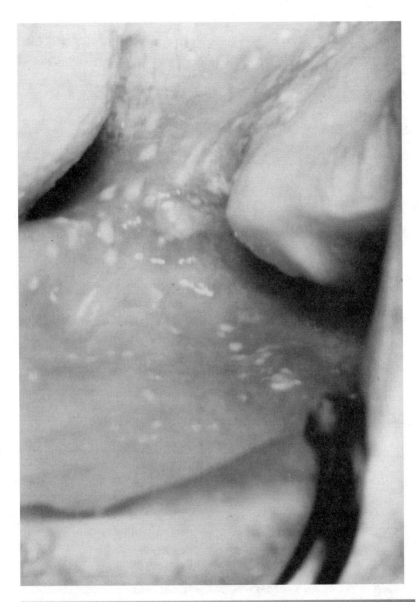

Figure 5-2

Oral *candidiasis*. The photograph shows the inside of the mouth, with the gums, cheek, and tongue (on the right). The white spots are areas of *Candida* (yeast) infection.

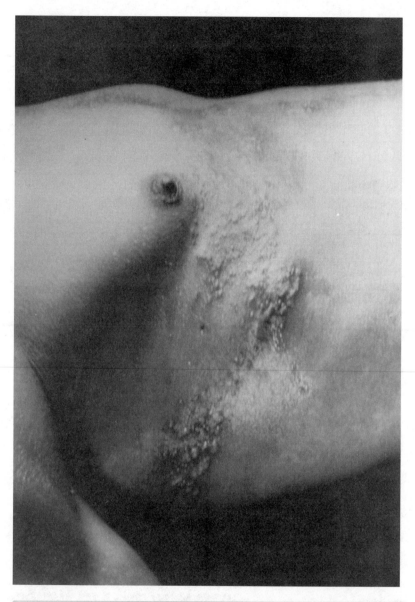

Figure 5–3

Shingles. Reactivation of the latent *Varicella zoster* (chicken pox virus) infection is shown in a band across the torso.

caused by the reactivation of a latent virus called *Varicella zoster*. This is the virus that causes chicken pox during childhood; it is a member of the Herpes virus family. After the initial childhood infection, the virus can remain dormant in the nerve trunks for many years and become reactivated when the immune system is compromised or stressed. With AIDS patients, the severity of shingles appears to be greater than that seen in non-AIDS patients, presumably because of their failing immune systems. The antiviral drug acyclovir is sometimes used to help control shingles.

Hairy leukoplakia. This is an abnormal condition of the mouth in which white plaques appear on the surface of the tongue. These plaques are not caused by the overgrowth of a fungus or bacteria, however. They are the abnormal growth of the papillae cells of the tongue; these plaques cannot be scraped off. These overgrown cells resemble cancer cells and appear to result from infection with another virus called *Epstein-Barr virus*. Epstein-Barr virus is also a member of the Herpes virus family and causes infectious mononucleosis in young adults. Hairy leukoplakia is a condition unique to AIDS patients.

Full-blown AIDS

As discussed elsewhere in this book (Chapter 4, pp. 64–68 and Chapter 6), most HIV-infected individuals will develop some of the symptoms associated with AIDS within eight to ten years after initial infection in the absence of antiviral treatments. The rate at which infected individuals develop symptoms may vary somewhat among different risk groups. For instance, hemophiliacs who were infected by transfusions or blood products may develop AIDS at a slower rate than do gay men who had high numbers of sexual partners. This may be influenced by the number and nature of other microorganisms (potential opportunistic infections) that these people encounter. The following infections and cancers seen in AIDS patients are indications that the immune system has undergone a catastrophic failure and can no longer prevent life-threatening infections or cancers.

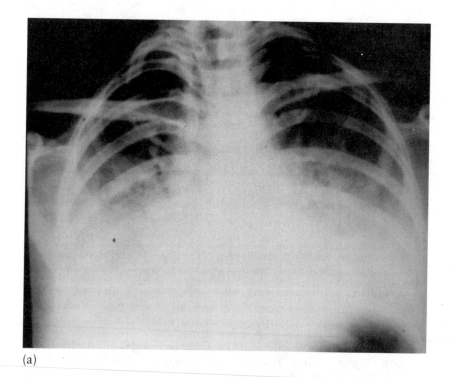

(a)

Figure 5–4

Pneumocystis carinii pneumonia. (a) A chest X-ray of an individual with PCP is shown. The ribs are apparent in the top of the X-ray, but they are not clear in the bottom. This is because the lungs inside the rib cage are filled with fluid, and they make that area of the X-ray appear lighter. In a normal individual, the ribs would be evident against a clear background at the bottom of the picture as well *(Courtesy of the Centers for Disease Control)*. (b) *Opposite.* Lung tissue from an individual with PCP. The dark round particles are *pneumocystis* microorganisms within the lung tissue.

Fungal Infections

***Pneumocystis carinii* pneumonia (PCP)**   This illness, which results from inflammation of the lungs, was originally the most common of the serious secondary infections seen with AIDS, and it has been a leading cause of death in AIDS patients. Inflamed areas of the lungs make them appear as white spots in lung X-rays (Figure 5–4). The inflammation is caused by infection with a fun-

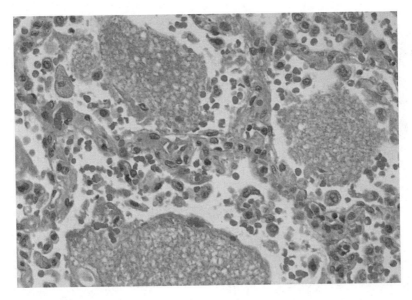

(b)

gus called *Pneumocystis carinii*. (Until recently, this microorganism was often classified as a protozoan, but it is now considered a fungus, based on molecular biological studies.) This microorganism gets its name from the person who discovered it, Carini, and from the fact that it can grow into cysts in the lungs of rats (pneumocystis). *Pneumocystis carinii* is relatively common, and small numbers of the fungus can be found in the lungs of healthy people as well as in many animals. It will cause disease in these animals if their immune systems are suppressed. In AIDS patients, the infection is often insidious, and the patient may be unaware of the seriousness of his or her illness. A dry cough is common, and a progressive shortness of breath indicates poor lung function. The shortness of breath is due to the inability of the inflamed lungs to take up adequate amounts of oxygen, which can lead to tissue damage throughout the body. *Pneumocystis carinii* particles are detected by staining the fluid washed out of the lungs with a special dye. PCP can be treated with various antibiotics called *sulfa drugs*. The antiparasitic agents trimethoprim and sulfamethoxazole (TMP-SMX) are usually given together to control the infection. Another drug called *pentamidine* is also used, especially when TMP-SMX becomes toxic to the patient. Although these antibiotic treatments are often successful, the lung infection can recur. Some drugs (Fancidar) may be given to prevent recurrences. New drugs, such as trimethexate (an anticancer drug), may also be effective against PCP.

Systemic mycosis   Three types of common soil fungi can cause generalized infections in AIDS patients. These fungi can exist in either a moldlike or a yeastlike form and are called *dimorphic*. The three types are *histoplasmosis, coccidiomycosis*, and *cryptococcus*. These fungi can cause lung infections in healthy people, but generalized or systemic infections are very rare. In AIDS patients, these fungi can cause devastating systemic infections that are massive and widespread. The brain, skin, bone, liver, and lymphatic tissue may all be highly infected. This will typically lead to death of the patient. Antifungal drugs such as miconazole are used to control these infections.

Protozoal Infections

Cryptosporidium **gastroenteritis**   This disease is caused by a protozoan called *cryptosporidium*. This protozoan infects the linings of the intestinal tract and causes diarrhea (gastroenteritis). In healthy people, diarrhea from a cryptosporidium infection is normally mild, lasting only a few days. However, in AIDS patients, the diarrhea is prolonged and severe. The AIDS patient may have from 20 to 50 watery stools per day, accompanied by abdominal cramps and profound weight loss. As a result, there is a serious loss of fluid and electrolytes (salts in the blood). Patients are treated with intravenous fluids and electrolytes, and their diarrhea can be controlled somewhat with drugs that slow intestinal action. However, currently no standard antibiotic is recognized for use against cryptosporidium. Spiramycin, which is an experimental drug, may help to control this persistent infection, but it does not eradicate it. Only about 5 percent of AIDS patients develop this disease. Cryptosporidium also infects cattle and other animals, especially their young; these animals may be the source of human infection.

Toxoplasmosis   This disease is caused by species of protozoa called *Toxoplasma gondii*, which normally causes an asymptomatic infection in healthy adults. This protozoan also infects a very wide variety of animals; domestic cats are one source of human infection. Unlike cryptosporidium, toxoplasma is an intracellular parasite and can invade numerous organs of infected individuals. In AIDS patients, the brain is often infected, which may result in symptoms similar to those seen with brain tumors: convulsions, disorientation, and dementia (Figure 5–5). A CT (computed tomography) scan is used to diagnose toxoplasmosis. Various antibiotics, such as pyrimethamine and sulfadiazine, are effective treatments, but they must be administered indefinitely to prevent a relapse. Unfortunately, some patients develop toxic reactions to these drugs.

Bacterial Infections

Interestingly, infections by commonly occurring bacteria (such as those in the lower intestines) do not generally occur in adult AIDS patients, perhaps because the components of the immune system responsible for controlling the common bacteria are less affected by HIV infection. However, children born infected with HIV often develop lung infections with common bacteria. In addition, adult AIDS patients may experience infections with tuberculosis-like bacteria.

Mycobacterium   This is a genus of bacteria that has characteristic cell walls with unusual staining properties in the laboratory. The bacterium that causes tuberculosis is a member of this genus. AIDS patients are most commonly infected with an atypical form of tuberculosis bacterium called *Mycobacterium avium-intracellulare*. This bacterium does not normally cause disease in healthy people, but in AIDS patients, it may cause a tuberculosis-like disease in the lungs. The infection can also involve numerous other tissues, such as the bone marrow, and bacteria may be present in the blood at very high levels (Figure 5–6). Patients with this opportunistic infection have fevers and low numbers of white blood cells. These infections are often resistant to drugs and are often treated with the simultaneous administration of up to six

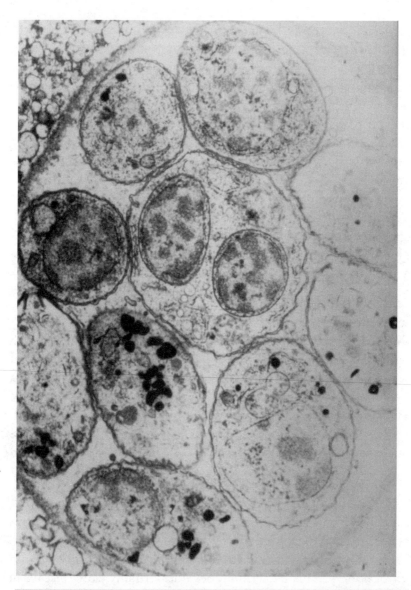

Figure 5–5

Toxoplasmosis. An electron microscope picture of a *toxoplasma* cyst is shown. A cyst is a walled-off area of microorganisms within a tissue. Each of the round areas in the photograph is a cross-section of a *toxoplasma* microorganism. *(Courtesy of the Centers for Disease Control)*

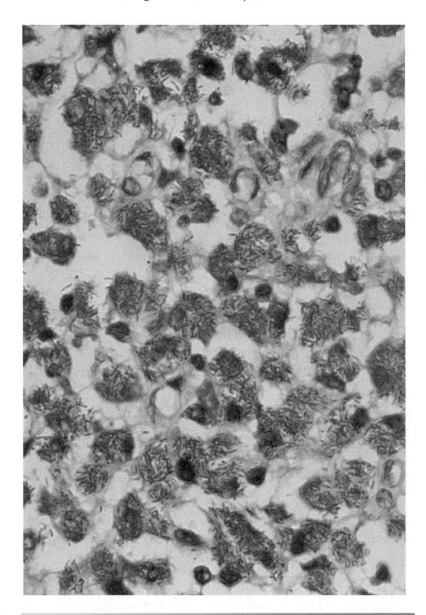

Figure 5–6

Mycobacterium avium-intracellularae infection of lymph node in a patient with AIDS. The small, dark rod-shaped particles are the mycobacterium. *(Courtesy of the Centers for Disease Control)*

different antibiotics. Isoniazid and rifampin are usually among the drugs used. This infection is more common in AIDS patients who were injection drug users.

More recently, standard tuberculosis (*Mycobacterium tuberculosis*) has become a common infection in AIDS patients. TB was largely eradicated in the United States by the mid-1970s through public health measures and antibiotic treatments. However, recently there has been a resurgence of TB, due to a combination of several factors: (1) increased immigration from areas where TB infection is still common (developing countries in Asia and Latin America); (2) a decline in funding for public health care measures, which has allowed TB to spread; and (3) AIDS patients, who are highly susceptible to TB infection and who in turn can transmit the bacterium. A very disturbing trend is the increasing appearance of TB strains that are resistant to antibiotics. This probably results from incomplete therapy of TB patients: To eradicate the bacteria a lengthy course of antibiotics is required, with repeated follow-up and testing until the bacteria are completely eliminated. However, if follow-up is incomplete, even if most of the TB bacteria are eliminated, the surviving bacteria can reestablish and spread to other individuals after antibiotic therapy is stopped. In addition, these bacteria are frequently resistant to the antibiotic that was administered. Tuberculosis is now a major threat to health-care workers, particularly in hospital settings where there are large numbers of indigent individuals, including AIDS patients.

Viral Infections

Cytomegalovirus   This is a member of the Herpes virus family, as are the Varicella zoster and Epstein-Barr viruses described earlier. Cytomegalovirus (CMV) is a common virus, and many people are infected early in childhood. Children tend to get an asymptomatic infection, whereas infected young adults may develop a mononucleosis-like illness. Infection of a fetus (a congenital infection) is very serious and can lead to permanent brain damage or death of the fetus. In AIDS patients, CMV infection can recur and tends to infect the retinas of eyes, leading to blindness. The virus also infects the adrenal gland, leading to hormonal imbalance. Pneumonia, fever, rash, and gastroenteritis due to CMV infection are also seen in AIDS patients. CMV pneumonia in patients who have PCP at the same time is usually fatal. The antiviral drug gancyclovir (related to acyclovir; see above) may help control CMV infections.

Cancers

Kaposi's sarcoma   Kaposi's sarcoma is tumors of the blood vessels (Figure 5–7). In non-AIDS patients, Kaposi's sarcoma (KS) is typically only seen in older men of Mediterranean or Jewish ancestry. In homosexual men with AIDS, up to 69 percent may develop Kaposi's sarcoma. Initially, only a few tumors appear as pink, purple, or brown skin lesions, usually located on the arms or legs. These tumors spread and become widely distributed, eventually involving most of the linings of the body. If they spread to the lungs, they are difficult to control. Chemotherapy can eradicate these tumors with a high success rate. Triaziquone, actinomycin D, bleomycin, and ICRF-159 are often used in

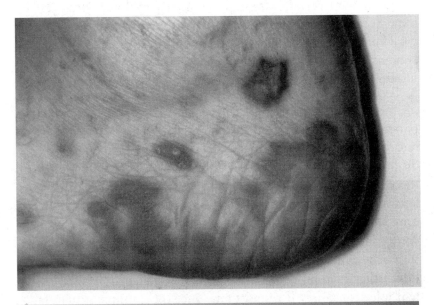

Figure 5–7

Kaposi's sarcoma. Dark (purplish) areas of Kaposi's sarcoma are shown on the heel of the foot.

chemotherapy. AIDS patients with KS often have a high level of opportunistic infections. Kaposi's sarcoma involves coinfection with another recently discovered member of the Herpes virus family (human herpes virus-8 [HHV8] or Kaposi's sarcoma herpesvirus [KSHV]).

Lymphomas   The lymphomas that occur in AIDS patients are cancers derived from the B-cells of the immune system. These are cells that make antibodies, as discussed in Chapter 3. Reactivation or coinfection in the B-lymphocytes with Epstein-Barr virus may be important for development of the lymphomas. As mentioned earlier in this chapter, the Epstein-Barr virus causes mononucleosis in young adults, but it can also transform normal B-cells into cancer cells. In AIDS patients, an unusual lymphoma that spreads to the brain also occurs.

Cervical Cancer   In female AIDS patients, cancer of the cervix (a part of the female genital tract) is also observed with high frequency. Cervical cancer is a fairly common cancer in women, although it typically affects women of middle age or older. Infection with certain strains of human papilloma virus (HPV) that cause warts in the genital tract is an underlying cause of cervical cancer. Like HIV, genital infection of HPV occurs by sexual contact. Thus, in AIDS patients, this HPV virus-induced cancer develops more rapidly in the absence of a normal immune system.

This list of opportunistic infections and cancers seen in AIDS patients covers only the most commonly observed diseases. Numerous other infections are also seen at lower frequencies. In addition, an individual patient may experience a combination of these illnesses. It is interesting that there are characteristic cancers and opportunistic infection in AIDS patients. These diseases are only a fraction of potential diseases that could affect an immunocompromised person. This may be due to the fact that HIV more seriously damages certain parts of the immune system. In addition, other factors, such as previously established chronic or latent infections, may be important. Once the immune system fails, the preexisting infectious agents can then proliferate and cause disease symptoms.

Different groups of HIV-infected individuals may differ in their symptoms. This may result from differing exposures to opportunistic agents, different ages, different sexes, or different geographical locations. For instance, in contrast to gay men, women with AIDS have a higher incidence of severe vaginal or oral yeast infections and cervical cancer; on the other hand, they rarely develop Kaposi's sarcoma. Children with AIDS suffer from more bacterial infections than do adult AIDS patients.

HIGH TURNOVER OF T$_{HELPER}$ CELLS IN AIDS PATIENTS

As described above, the immunological deficiency in AIDS patients results from the very low numbers of T$_{helper}$ cells present. The low number of T$_{helper}$ cells results from continual high-level destruction by viral infection. Even in an AIDS patient with very low numbers of T$_{helper}$ cells, the immune system produces many T$_{helper}$cells every day. However, the production of new T$_{helper}$ cells cannot keep up with the destruction of T$_{helper}$ cells brought on by HIV. It is estimated that an AIDS patient loses about two billion T$_{helper}$ cells every day and that his/her immune system is making almost the same number every day in an attempt to replenish them.

ANTIVIRAL DRUG TREATMENTS IN AIDS

To restore the health of an AIDS patient, it is necessary to suppress replication of HIV and to rebuild the damaged immune system (see Chapter 8). So far, antiviral drugs have played the most important part in the clinical treatment of this disease.

AZT And Other Nucleoside Analogs

AZT was the first drug to show benefit in treatment of AIDS patients, and it is still one of the primary drugs in use (see Chapters 4 and 6). AIDS patients who are given AZT show increased survival. Without AZT, the average life expectancy of an AIDS patient who has an opportunistic infection is about six months. With AZT, that life expectancy rises to one and one-half years.

Treatment with AZT actually results in some recovery of immune function. The number of T_{helper} lymphocytes in AZT-treated AIDS patients increases; they experience fewer opportunistic infections, and they may actually gain weight. The patients also feel better. Although AZT is rarely used by itself anymore (see Combination Therapies, p. 106), we first discuss its use as a "monotherapy," because this was the original way it was used.

The cost of AZT is high—about $3,500 per year for one person. The original treatment regimen demanded that a patient take an AZT pill once every four hours, around the clock. As mentioned in Chapter 4, AZT treatment has some side effects, such as nausea, headache, and loss of sleep. The major complication is that about half of treated patients become anemic and have a low white blood cell count. This in itself can lead to an increase in bacterial infections. If anemia occurs, AZT treatment must be discontinued, at least temporarily.

The success of AZT in treating patients with clinical AIDS led to the practice of treating asymptomatic HIV-infected individuals. Preliminary studies in the late 1980s indicated that AZT treatment of these people slowed the rate of decline of their immune systems. Moreover, some of the toxic side effects (anemia) occurred less frequently. This led to the general recommendation that individuals who suspect that they may have been exposed to HIV be tested (under conditions that ensure counseling and confidentiality). If they were infected, their immune systems could then be monitored for signs of damage (e.g., T_{helper} lymphocyte counts; see Chapter 4), and opportunistic infections could be monitored as well. Preventive therapies such as AZT and aerosol pentamidine (to prevent PCP) could then be used before the individual became seriously ill. Seriously ill patients are much more difficult to treat medically. As we shall see below (under combination therapies), these recommendations have been modified recently.

In the mid-1990s, the advisability of treating asymptomatic HIV-infected individuals with AZT was called into question by a large clinical trial (the Concorde trial) held in England and France. In this study, asymptomatic HIV-infected individuals were treated with AZT and compared with a matched group, who received no drug. There was no difference in the rate of AIDS-related deaths between the AZT-treated and untreated individuals. The limited effectiveness of AZT in asymptomatic individuals is related to the development of AZT-resistant virus (see below). It is important to remember that even if the value of treating asymptomatic individuals with AZT is unclear, the drug clearly has a positive effect in extending and improving the quality of life in AIDS patients if it is administered for the first time to individuals after they have developed symptoms (see Table 6–5).

As mentioned in Chapter 4, AZT is a *nucleoside analog.* Four other nucleoside analog drugs have also been approved for treatment of HIV-infected individuals and AIDS patients: *dideoxyinosine (DDI), dideoxycytidine (DDC), 3TC (lamivudine), and D4T (stavudine)* (see Table 5–1). All of these drugs are analogs of DNA building blocks that terminate further DNA synthesis if incorporated into DNA by HIV reverse transcriptase. DDI has been approved as an alternative drug for HIV-infected individuals who cannot tolerate AZT. DDC has been approved for use in combination with AZT, as has D4T. Side effects are also problems with these drugs. For instance, some individuals taking DDI develop pancreatitis (a serious inflammation of the pancreas), and some individuals on DDC experience peripheral neuropathies (tingling in the extremities).

Development of Drug-resistant HIV

As discussed in Chapter 4, pp. 74–76, development of drug-resistance in HIV-infected individuals taking antiviral drugs is the major limitation of their effectiveness. HIV has an unusually high mutation rate. During the many cycles of viral replication in an infected individual, a mutated virus with an altered reverse transcriptase will be produced that does not efficiently incorporate AZT into HIV DNA. As a result, in HIV-infected individuals who have been taking AZT, there is a selection process for AZT-resistant virus. Once AZT-resistant HIV becomes the predominant virus in the infected individual, AZT treatment does not provide any benefit.

The viral RNA load assays described in Chapter 4 allow us to see how serious the problem of drug resistance is for HIV antivirals. When an HIV-infected individual first begins to take AZT,

Table 5–1
CURRENTLY APPROVED HIV ANTIVIRAL DRUGS

Drug Class	Chemical/Generic Name	Trade Name
Nucleoside analogs		
	AZT/azidothymidine/ zidovudine	Retrovir
	DDI/dideoxyinosine/ didanosine	Videx
	DDC/dideoxycytidine/ zalcitabine	HIVID
	3TC/lamivudine	Epivir
	D4T/stavudine	Zerit
Non-nucleoside reverse transcriptase inhibitors (NRTIs)		
	Nevirapine	Viramune
	Delavirdine	Rescriptor
	Abacavir	Ziagen
Protease inhibitors		
	Saquinavir	Fortovase
	Indinavir	Crixivan
	Ritonavir	Norvir
	Nelfinavir	Viracept
	Amprenavir	Agenerase

there is usually a 10- to 100-fold drop in the amount of HIV RNA circulating in the blood. However, within a year, the amount of viral RNA in the blood returns to nearly the same level as before drug treatment began. Moreover, the HIV is AZT-resistant. This may explain why AZT treatment of asymptomatic individuals has limited benefit—for the treatment to be effective, it has to suppress viral replication for many years.

Drug resistance has been a problem with every HIV antiviral drug developed so far. For instance, as described above for AZT, treatment with all of the nucleoside analog compounds leads to development of drug-resistant virus (with drug-resistant reverse transcriptase). However, the changes in amino acid building blocks that lead to an AZT-resistant reverse transcriptase may be different from changes in reverse transcriptase resistant to another drug (e.g., 3TC). As a result, an HIV that is resistant to AZT is often sensitive to inhibition by 3TC. Thus, long-term treatment of HIV-infected individuals involves rotating them onto new antiviral drugs as their virus becomes resistant to those they are currently taking. Continued development of more HIV antiviral drugs will be important.

AZT Treatment of Pregnant Women

AZT treatment alone has had an important effect on preventing transmission of HIV infection from pregnant women to their children. HIV-infected pregnant women have about a 23 percent chance of transmitting infection to their offspring. Treating women with AZT during pregnancy lowers the risk for transmitting infection to the newborn by 70 percent. Thus, AZT treatment is now recommended for pregnant women. This is one of the few currently recommended uses of AZT monotherapy.

Non-nucleoside Inhibitors of Reverse Transcriptase

Other drugs that target the HIV reverse transcriptase are also under development. In particular, drugs that bind to the reverse transcriptase enzyme and prevent it from functioning have been developed. These are called *non-nucleoside of reverse transcriptase inhibitors (NRTIs)* (Table 5–1). One such drug, nevirapine, was approved for treatment in 1996. Nevirapine has some advantages: it has relatively few side effects, and it leads to even better initial decreases in viral RNA load than do the nucleoside analogs—1000- to 10,000-fold decreases. However, nevirapine-resistant HIV arises quickly in infected individuals who are taking the drug. In 1997, a second non-nucleoside reverse transcriptase inhibitor, delavirdane, was approved for use, and a third (abacavir) has also been recently approved.

Recently, a single dose of nevirapine has been shown to be effective in substantially reducing HIV transmission from pregnant women to their children. This is much cheaper and simpler than AZT monotherapy (see preceding section) and is particularly promising for the developing world, where continual treatment of pregnant women with AZT through their pregnancy may not be affordable.

Protease Inhibitors

Protease inhibitors are the newest and currently most effective class of HIV antiviral drugs. The role of protease in maturation of virus particles is discussed in Chapter 4, p. 76. Protease inhibitors bind to the HIV protease and inhibit its activity. Four HIV protease inhibitors have been approved for use: saquinavir, ritonavir, indinivir, and nelfinavir (see Table 5–1). The protease inhibitors have some advantages when given to patients: very strong initial decreases in viral RNA load (1000- to 10,000-fold decreases) and relatively few side effects. However, in patients receiving only a protease inhibitor, resistant HIV develops rapidly. Moreover, the drug-resistant virus often shows cross-resistance to other protease inhibitors. For instance, HIV that is resistant to indinavir is generally resistant to ritonavir as well. Thus, once an HIV-infected person taking a protease inhibitor develops drug-resistant virus, it is likely that other protease inhibitors will be of limited benefit.

The protease inhibitors have been most effective when used in combination therapies.

Combination Therapies

The use of drug combinations in treatment of many human diseases is well established. The treatment of cancer, another long-term disease, is a good example. Chemotherapy (drug treatment) for cancer became effective only after the development of drug combinations. At the maximum tolerable doses of one chemotherapy drug, most of the cancer cells in a patient may be killed, but a noticeable fraction will survive—typically one in 100 or one in 1,000. Those surviving cells will grow back and lead to recurrence of the tumor. However, if a second chemotherapeutic drug is combined with the first drug, the second drug can cause further killing of the tumor cells that survive the first drug. In practice, by the time three or four drugs are combined in a successful chemotherapy cocktail, they can lead to complete eradication of the tumor cells in the cancer patient.

Development of combination antiviral therapies for HIV-infected individuals has been under way for several years. The first combination therapies involved combinations of two nucleoside analogs, since those were the first drugs available. Clinical trials showed that combined treatment of HIV-infected patients with AZT and DDC provided some benefit in comparison to treatment with either drug alone. Another noteworthy combination was AZT with 3TC. Laboratory experiments suggested that, although HIV can mutate to resistance to either AZT or 3TC alone, it has difficulty mutating into a virus whose reverse transcriptase is resistant to both AZT and 3TC. Thus, combination antiviral therapy may provide a solution to the development of drug resistance in HIV-infected people.

The development of the protease inhibitors has led to some extremely effective combination therapies for HIV-infected individuals. Currently, the most effective combinations involve the use of two nucleoside analogs and one protease inhibitor. For example, one combination is the nucleoside analogs AZT and 3TC along with the protease inhibitor indinavir. These combinations are sometimes referred to as *"triple combination therapies"* or *"AIDS drug cocktails"* or "HAART" (highly active antiretroviral therapy). The triple combination therapies are much more potent than the previous single-drug treatments. For instance, in the triple combination of AZT plus 3TC plus indinavir, a majority of HIV-infected people experience a drop in viral RNA loads in the blood to below the level of detectability. Moreover, this effect has been sustained for several years. In general, the drops in viral RNA loads in the blood have been accompanied by recoveries of T_{helper} cell counts (in some cases very dramatic), and increases in immune function and in the disappearance of AIDS symptoms.

The development of the triple combination therapies has led to a new approach for managing HIV-infected individuals. Since the viral RNA loads during the asymptomatic period predict the rate of progression to clinical AIDS, some medical doctors now believe that the best strategy is to aggressively treat asymptomatic people with a triple combination of antiviral drugs right away. This reduces or eliminates the viral RNA loads during the asymptomatic period. Regular monitoring for viral RNA loads should be carried out, and adjustments or changes in the combination therapies should be made if the viral RNA loads begin to climb. It is hoped that this approach will substantially delay or halt the progression of HIV-infected people to AIDS.

Limitations and Uncertainties in the Triple Combination (HAART) Therapies

The dramatic successes with the introduction of the protease inhibitors and triple combination therapies received a great deal of attention in the press. Some news stories at the time suggested that the threat of AIDS was over and that it may be possible to "cure" people of HIV infection. These stories were premature. It is important to remember that the protease inhibitors and triple combination therapies were introduced only in 1996. Although the initial effects have been very promising, it will take many years before we will know the true value of these drugs in inhibiting or slowing the progression of HIV infection. As discussed earlier in this chapter, the average latency for progression of HIV infection to clinical AIDS is approximately eight to ten years. It will take us at least that long to learn if the triple combination therapies are effective in preventing progression to AIDS.

Here are some specific limitations or uncertainties about the current combination therapies:

1. *The triple combination therapies are not effective in all people.* Although the triple combination therapies have had remarkable benefits for many HIV-infected individuals, they have not been as effective for others. For some people, viral RNA loads in the blood have not shown very large decreases, or they have shown only temporary decreases. The triple combination therapies generally are less effective for HIV-infected individuals who have previously taken antiviral drugs (e.g., AZT or other nucleoside analogs). This is because such individuals generally already harbor significant levels of HIV that is resistant to the nucleoside analogs (see above). As a result, in these people, the triple combination

therapies are, effectively, more like single therapy with a protease inhibitor; as mentioned above, protease-resistant HIV rapidly appears in individuals taking protease inhibitors alone.

2. *Uncertainty about the duration of effectiveness.* Because the triple combination therapies were introduced only in 1996, we do not yet know how long they will be effective in an HIV-infected person. The current results are encouraging, but it has yet to be determined if any of the triple combination therapies will be able to suppress viral RNA loads over the long term. In fact, in extended clinical trials, the percentages of infected people who show complete suppression of viral RNA loads from a particular triple combination thereapy decrease. HIV mutants that are resistant to all drugs in a triple combination therapy are now appearing in patient populations.

3. *Drug side effects.* As discussed earlier in this chapter, several of the HIV antivirals have side effects (particularly the nucleoside analogs). This is a particular problem because HIV-infected individuals may need lifelong antiviral treatment. As a result, even relatively minor side effects may become serious after prolonged treatment. Part of the challenge for doctors managing HIV-infected patients is to find new triple combinations, if the patients can no longer tolerate the side effects of one triple combination. While the protease inhibitors have generally shown fewer side effects, prolonged treatment has resulted in an unusual (but not life-threatening) one: redistribution of body fat to unusual locations such as the back of the neck.

4. *Difficulty in maintaining treatment schedules.* Taking the triple combination therapies is a very complex matter. In a typical triple combination therapy, an individual may need to take as many as twenty-five pills per day at very precise intervals. Individuals must faithfully take the different drugs at the prescribed times in order to keep the proper levels of drugs in their systems. Moreover, some of the protease inhibitors have very specific requirements for administration. For instance, the protease inhibitor indinavir must be taken on an empty stomach. The protease inhibitor ritonavir seriously affects the metabolism of other drugs that are used in the therapy of AIDS patients. This presents a serious chal-

lenge for doctors who are treating AIDS patients, as well as to the patients themselves.

In the triple combination therapies, strict adherence to the treatment regimen is very important. It has been found that if patients receive doses of protease inhibitor that are not optimal, this can actually accelerate the rate of development of protease inhibitor–resistant HIV. As mentioned above, once a resistant HIV has developed, it is often resistant to other protease inhibitors as well. Maintaining *treatment adherence* is a major concern for physicians and AIDS health-care workers. This is a particular challenge for HIV-infected individuals who already have difficult access to health care—for instance, economically disadvantaged people or injection drug users.

5. *Cost.* The triple combination therapies are very expensive. As discussed earlier in this chapter, the cost of AZT treatment alone is about $3,500 per year for a patient. Each drug in a triple combination costs at least that much; the current annual cost of a triple combination therapy is about $15,000 per person. If we consider that there are between 500,000 and 1,000,000 people in the United States who are living with HIV infection, it would take $8–15 billion yearly to provide triple combination therapies to all of them. This is clearly a serious challenge to our health-care system. We should also consider that worldwide, most of the cases of HIV infection and AIDS are in developing countries (see Chapter 6). These countries do not yet have the financial resources to provide triple combination therapies to their infected populations.

Recently, concerns about the duration of the effectiveness of the triple combination therapies have increased. Initially, introduction of HAART therapy led to a striking decrease in both the rates of AIDS deaths and also in the appearance of new AIDS cases (see Figure 6–1 and 8–1 and Table 8–2). However, the most recent numbers indicate a marked slowing in the decrease of new AIDS cases and AIDS deaths. This apears to reflect development of drug-resistant virus, drug side effects, and difficulties in treatment adherence. This underlines the importance of developing new and better anti-HIV drugs and also of developing effective measures to prevent new infections.

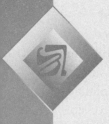

CHAPTER 6
Epidemiology and AIDS

In the preceding chapter, we considered how HIV manifests itself in an infected individual. The next level of complexity is to consider how HIV moves between individuals and its effects on populations. For these topics, the discipline of epidemiology is very important. This chapter gives an overview of epidemiology, with some applications regarding HIV and AIDS. The modes of HIV transmission and relative risk factors are addressed in Chapter 7.

Epidemiology is the study of the patterns of disease occurrence in populations and of the factors affecting them. This field is of great importance to the understanding of human diseases, and epidemiological studies can be used to address many questions. Epidemiological studies can:

- *identify new diseases*
- *identify populations at risk for a disease*
- *identify possible causative agents of a disease*
- *identify factors or behaviors that increase risk of a disease and also determine the relative importance of a factor in contributing to a disease*
- *rule out factors or behaviors as contributing to a disease*
- *evaluate therapies for a disease*
- *guide the development of effective public health measures and preventive strategies.*

It is important to keep in mind that epidemiological studies involve large groups or *populations* of individuals. This approach gives great power to these studies, since they draw on the total experience and behavior of large numbers of individuals.

Because epidemiological studies are based on observation of groups, some limitations and risks in interpretations are introduced. One limitation is that these studies cannot predict how any single individual will be affected by a factor even if the population as a whole is affected by that factor. Epidemiological studies also cannot predict the course a disease will take in a particular person. Some risks are associated with drawing improper conclusions from epidemiology. For instance, it is important to avoid making an ecological fallacy: explaining behavior of an individual based on observations of an entire group. Another example of an improper conclusion is identifying certain characteristics of a group as causing a disease. For example, epidemiological studies have identified male homosexuals as one of the groups at high risk for AIDS. This does not imply that simply being homosexual causes AIDS, as some people have claimed. Instead, certain sexual behaviors by some gay men link them to AIDS, as we shall see later in this chapter and also in Chapter 7.

Despite these limitations and risks, epidemiological studies provide some of the most definitive information about the causes and dynamics of human diseases, short of carrying out experiments on humans.

AN OVERVIEW OF EPIDEMIOLOGY AND AIDS

Epidemiology has played a central role in the fight against AIDS right from the beginning, and this will continue. The initial identification of AIDS as a new syndrome in 1981 was made through epidemiological studies. These studies reported the unusually high occurrence of individuals with rare diseases associated with immunological defects (see Chapter 1). The initial epidemiological studies showed a high frequency of the new disease in sexually active male homosexuals. Furthermore, the pattern of occurrence suggested that AIDS might be caused by an infectious agent that could be transmitted by sexual means. Subsequently, the appearance of AIDS cases among recipients of blood transfusions or blood products (for instance, hemophiliacs) as well as injection drug users suggested that AIDS could be transmitted through contaminated blood. The study of individuals afflicted with AIDS and also of groups of high-risk individuals led to the isolation in 1984 of HIV, the virus that causes AIDS. As soon as HIV was isolated, the virus was used to develop the test for HIV antibodies (see Chapter 4, p. 68). The availability of the HIV antibody test allowed much more accurate epidemiological studies because evidence of infection could also be detected in healthy asymptomatic individuals. This led to the realization that an alarming number of individuals have been infected with HIV in many parts of the world. Moreover, we are currently seeing only the tip of the HIV iceberg, since it often takes several years for the disease to develop. Epidemiological studies of high-risk groups have identified the underlying high-risk behaviors, such as unprotected sexual intercourse and sharing IV needles. This, in turn, has led to development of public health measures and safe-sex guidelines, which are our only weapons in AIDS prevention today. Finally, epidemiological studies (which also could be classified as clinical studies) provided the proof that azidothymidine (AZT) is an effective therapeutic drug for AIDS.

BASIC CONCEPTS IN EPIDEMIOLOGY

The two basic kinds of epidemiological studies are *descriptive* and *analytical*. The goal of the first is to describe the occurrence of disease in populations. Analytical studies seek to identify and explain the causes of diseases. Frequently, descriptive epidemiological studies lead to analytical studies. For instance, descriptive epidemiology may identify a new disease, such as AIDS, or suggest hypotheses about the causes of a disease. Interpretation of the descriptive studies will then suggest hypotheses leading to analytical studies that examine the disease in more detail.

Since epidemiology is the study of disease in populations, the proportion of affected individuals in a population is of basic importance. There are two important measures used in epidemiology:

Prevalence. This is the fraction (or proportion) of current living individuals in a population who have a disease or infection at a particular time.

Incidence. This is the proportion of a population that develops *new* cases of a disease or infection during a particular time period.

As an example, let's look at Table 6–1. It shows the number of individuals with evidence of previous infection with hepatitis B virus (antibodies for the virus) in a city for the years 1968 and 1988. During this time, the population of the city has increased

Table 6–1
HEPATITIS B VIRUS INFECTION IN A CITY*

	1968	1988
Total population	100,000	150,000
Individuals with hepatitis B virus antibodies (seropositives)	500	1,000
Prevalence of seropositive individuals	0.5% (500/100,000)	0.67% (1,000/150,000)

*This is an example for discussion only. Three different viruses can actually cause hepatitis.

from 100,000 to 150,000. The *prevalence* of hepatitis B virus infection was 0.5 percent in 1968, and it increased to 0.67 percent in 1988. The *incidence* of infection during this period was 0.17 percent (0.67 percent minus 0.5 percent); put another way, there were 170 new cases of infection per 100,000 people during the 20-year period. The *yearly* incidence rate would be 0.17 percent divided by 20 (0.0085 percent new cases per 100,000 people per year). Epidemiologists use these prevalence and incidence data to calculate other expressions of their results, such as risk values.

Descriptive Studies

Descriptive epidemiological studies measure the appearance of disease by categories of *person*, *place*, and *time*. An example of disease appearance by person is the observation that lung cancer predominantly appears in individuals who smoke cigarettes (*person* = smokers). Disease appearance by place, for example, would be studies showing the low incidence of tooth decay in areas where there is a high level of naturally occurring fluorides in the water supply (*place* = high-fluoride areas). Disease appearance by time might be an outbreak of food poisoning resulting from contaminated food at a picnic (*time* = days after the picnic).

An important concept in descriptive epidemiology is clustering. *Clustering* is the unusually high incidence *or* prevalence of a disease in a subpopulation. Clustering can occur by person, place, time, or a combination. The first documented outbreak of Legionnaire's disease is a good example of clustering. Legionnaire's disease is a serious bacterial respiratory infection that can be fatal if untreated. The disease was first identified among several members of the American Legion who attended an American Legion convention at a hotel in Philadelphia in the summer of 1976. Thus, the disease was clustered with respect to place (the hotel in Philadelphia), time (1976), and person (American Legion members). Ultimately, a new microorganism (*Legionella*) was isolated, which causes Legionnaire's disease.

Types of Descriptive Epidemiological Studies

Descriptive epidemiological studies are carried out according to several design strategies or a combination of these strategies. Two of the important strategies are *case reports/case report series* and *cross-sectional/prevalence studies*.

Case reports/case report series   *Case reports* are descriptions of an unusual disease occurrence in individual patients. Sometimes the nature of the case may also suggest a relationship between some predisposing factor and the disease, or it may suggest the appearance of a new disease. These suggestions are strengthened if several similar cases are observed and reported together—a *case report series*. The original report in 1981 by Gottlieb describing pneumocystis pneumonia in six homosexual men is a classic example of a case report series (see Chapter 1). This report suggested that a new disease (AIDS) might be occurring and that male homosexuals were at high risk.

Cross-sectional/prevalence studies   In these studies, a population is monitored for the occurrence of a disease or a series of diseases, and statistics about each case (nature of the patient, geographical location) are recorded. This information can be used to construct a cross-sectional profile for the disease or diseases within the population. These studies are also sometimes carried out over a long period of time, and the date of disease occurrence is also recorded. Once the cross-sectional profile is obtained, then it can be examined for clustering of disease cases by person, place, or time. These clusterings can suggest causes of known diseases and also identify new ones.

Cancer registries are an example of these studies. In these registries, information is gathered about all cases of cancer occurring in a region. Information from the cancer registry can then be used by cancer epidemiologists to investigate potential causes of cancer. For instance, these registries have provided strong evidence for a causal relationship between cigarette smoking and lung cancer.

The United States Public Health Service Centers for Disease Control (CDC) maintains a registry of deaths and diseases, which is reported on a weekly basis in a journal called *Morbidity and Mortality Weekly Report*. Information from this registry was also important in characterizing the AIDS epidemic in 1981 and 1982, since there was a sharp increase in cases of pneumocystis pneumonia and Kaposi's sarcoma at that time. The CDC now publishes a regular HIV/AIDS surveillance report that provides current and past epidemiological information exclusively on HIV infection and AIDS (see Appendix).

Prevalence studies can also be used to identify groups within the population that are at higher risk for a particular disease. In addition to suggesting possible causes of the disease, this information can be used for other purposes. First, if the disease is rare in the overall population, it will be more efficient to study the disease by focusing on the high-risk population—this is important for analytical epidemiology (see below). Second, public health workers may want to focus particular attention on the high-risk population as a first step in working out prevention strategies to combat the disease.

Analytical Studies

Analytical epidemiology studies are generally more focused than are descriptive studies. They investigate the causes of a particular disease, and they often involve assigning a numerical value to (quantifying) a potential risk factor. In fact, the distinction between descriptive and analytical studies is not absolute. Most epidemiological studies fall somewhere between a completely descriptive study and a purely analytical one. For instance, cancer registries can be used for analytical epidemiology studies, in which the relationship between a particular factor and a disease (for instance, smoking and lung cancer) is examined in detail, and the relative risk is determined.

Types of Analytical Epidemiological Studies

The two main approaches to analytical epidemiology are *experimental/interventional studies* and *observational studies*.

Experimental/interventional studies In these studies, a condition of an experimental subpopulation is changed, and the effect on the development of a disease is observed. The results are compared with the main population or an untreated subpopulation. This approach has been very useful in testing potential therapies for diseases. For instance, the Salk polio vaccine was tested in a nationwide trial of second- and third-grade school children in 1953–1954. The success of the trial led to the acceptance of the vaccine and the elimination of polio as a major health threat. A more recent example is a test of a vaccine for hepatitis B virus. This vaccine was tested in a population of sexually active male homosexuals (who are also at high risk for hepatitis B infection) and was shown to be very effective. Clinical drug trials can also be considered interventional epidemiology.

Although interventional studies are very useful in testing therapies, it is often difficult to use them to directly test if a factor causes a disease. Treating a group of people with a factor that might cause a disease raises serious ethical questions. This is particularly important if, as is the case for AIDS, there is no effective treatment or cure for the disease. One possible solution to this dilemma is to see if the same disease can be induced by the factor in animals. Another approach is observational epidemiology.

Observational studies Observational studies take advantage of the fact that, within a population, certain individuals will encounter a factor and develop a disease but others will not. The epidemiologist does not change the conditions of people to study the disease but rather *subdivides* the population according to possible risk factors or disease and studies them separately. For instance, by subdividing a population into cigarette smokers and nonsmokers, the epidemiologist can investigate the effect of cigarette smoking on cancer or heart disease without making anybody smoke. In some cases, a properly designed observational study can provide the same information as an interventional study.

The two main types of observational studies are: *case/control studies* and *cohort studies.*

Case/control studies involve studying a group of individuals with a particular disease (the cases) and comparing them with a group of unaffected individuals (the controls). The controls are often matched for a number of factors not believed to be involved in the disease. If the cases differ from the controls by another factor as well, this would suggest that the factor is related to the disease. For instance, if lung cancer patients are compared to individuals without lung cancer, a higher percentage of the cancer patients are cigarette smokers than in the control population.

Case/control studies are particularly useful if the disease being studied occurs only rarely. For instance, if a disease occurs only once per million people in the United States, it would be impractical to survey everybody in the population to study those few cases that occur. On the other hand, nationally, there would be about 200 cases of the disease, which could be readily studied by the case/control approach. For the same reason, case/control studies are important at the beginning of infectious disease epidemics, when there are still very few cases. The early epidemiology studies in the AIDS epidemic were mainly case/control studies.

Cohort studies focus on a group of individuals who share a particular risk factor for a disease. This group is then examined for the frequency or rate of disease appearance in comparison to a control population that does not have the risk factor. Such studies can implicate or exonerate a potential risk factor for the disease, and they can also determine the degree to which the risk factor contributes to the disease.

Cohort studies can go forward or backward in time. *Prospective* cohort studies go forward in time, starting with an identified cohort of individuals and documenting development of disease as time progresses. A number of cohort studies for AIDS have been carried out, principally involving gay or bisexual men. For instance, one cohort study involved HIV antibody-positive individuals and tracked occurrence of lymphadenopathy syndrome (LAS), ARC, and AIDS. In another study, a group of single men in San Francisco are being followed for infection with HIV, and the factors (sexual practices, injection drug use) associated with infection are being studied.

Cohort studies that go back in time are called *retrospective* studies. In these studies, exposure to the risk factor has occurred previously, and the cohort of individuals is later identified for observation. For instance, retrospective cohort studies have been carried out on individuals who worked in asbestos-processing plants in the 1940s and 1950s. These individuals subsequently showed a high incidence of lung cancer, implicating asbestos as another potential cause of lung cancer.

Correlations

In analytical epidemiology, results are considered in terms of *statistical associations* or *correlations* between a factor and a disease. For instance, a high frequency of cigarette smoking is found among lung cancer patients, which means there is a statistical association between cigarette smoking and lung cancer. The aim of analytical epidemiology is to deduce *causality* from the statistical association, in our example, that cigarette smoking causes lung cancer. However, statistical associations have other possible explanations.

Three possible reasons for a positive correlation between a factor and a disease are:

1. *There is no causal relationship.* This could result from faulty design of the experiment. For instance, if the control population is not properly matched with the experimental population, a false correlation could be observed.

2. *There is an indirect relationship.* In some situations a third *confounding* variable may influence both the factor being tested and the disease. For instance, there is a positive statistical correlation between alcohol consumption and lung cancer, but this does not mean that alcohol causes lung cancer. In this case, cigarette smoking is a confounding variable.

Cigarette smoking causes lung cancer, *and* cigarette smoking is statistically associated with alcohol consumption. That is, individuals who are cigarette smokers also tend to drink more alcohol than do nonsmokers.

Another example of an indirect relationship is the high statistical correlation between swimsuit sales and ice cream sales. This does not mean that ice cream consumption leads to swimsuit purchases or vice versa. In this case, summer or high temperature is a confounding variable. More swimsuits are bought during the summer when it is warm and beach weather is good, and more people eat ice cream during this time because it is hot.

3. *There is a direct causal relationship.* That is, a change in the factor will lead to a change in occurrence of the disease. It is important to remember that more than one factor can be a direct cause of a disease. Thus, establishment of a direct causal relationship between one factor and a disease does not rule out other factors as well.

Criteria for a Causal Relationship

In observational studies, it is difficult to absolutely prove a causal relationship from a correlation because the epidemiologist does not change the factors under study. However, certain criteria provide tests for causality. They are:

1. *Strength of the association* between the factor and the disease. The strongest correlation would be if everybody with the factor gets the disease, and nobody without the factor gets the disease. A strong correlation makes a causal relationship more likely. The argument is also strengthened if there is a dose-response relationship—that is, if individuals who have received higher exposure to a factor show higher frequencies of disease. However, it is always important to keep in mind that confounding variables could exist.

2. *The association is consistent;* that is, if the same correlation is observed in other studies, using different settings and different populations.

3. *The association has the correct time relationship;* that is, exposure to the agent must occur *before* development of the disease.

4. *The association has biological plausibility;* that is, association of the factor with the disease makes biological sense.

For infectious agents, another set of rules has been developed for assessing whether a microbe causes a disease: *Koch's
postulates.* Koch's postulates are discussed in Chapter 2, p. 16,
and they require both observational and experimental studies.
Briefly, a microorganism can be considered the cause of a disease
if (1) it is always found in diseased individuals, (2) it can be isolated from a diseased individual and grown pure in culture, (3)
the pure microorganism can cause the disease when introduced
into susceptible individuals, and (4) the same microorganism can
be reisolated from those individuals.

EPIDEMIOLOGY AND AIDS IN THE UNITED STATES

Let us now see what epidemiology can tell us about AIDS in more
detail. As described in the overview to this chapter, epidemiology
has been extremely important in this epidemic. Let's look at some
of the epidemiological information and the conclusions that can
be drawn from it.

The Current Picture of AIDS in the United States

Figure 6–1 shows the total number of AIDS cases that have been
reported in the United States for the years 1978 through 1997. By
the end of 1997, a total of 641,086 cases had been reported, of
which 390,084 had died. Current estimates are that between
650,000 and 900,000 people in the United States are infected
with HIV; many of these people may develop AIDS and ultimately
die if the new therapies are not completely effective. Thus, we can
see the seriousness of this epidemic and the strain that it will place
on our society.

Figure 6–2 shows the distribution of AIDS cases according
to risk groups. Homosexual and bisexual men make up the
largest percentage of cases, followed by injection drug users, hemophiliacs and recipients of blood transfusions, sexual partners
of HIV-infected individuals, and children of HIV-infected moth-

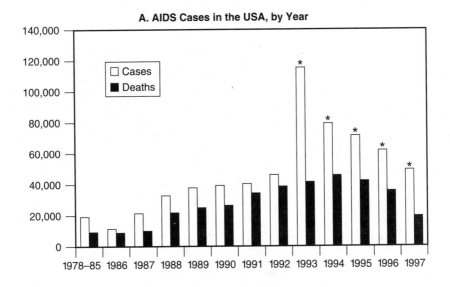

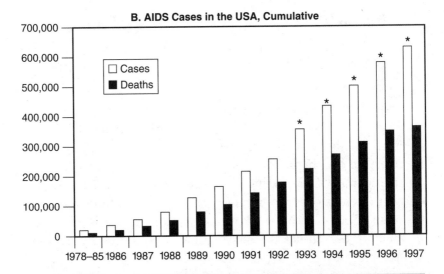

Figure 6–1

Appearance of AIDS in the USA. Data compiled from the December 1998 HIV/AIDS Surveillance Report from the U.S. Centers for Disease Control. In 1993, the definition for AIDS was expanded to include any HIV-positive person with a T_{helper} count of less than 200 per cubic millimeter of blood. This accounts for the jump in the number of reported AIDS cases beginning in 1993. Data for all subsequent years use this new definition (designated by * on the graphs).

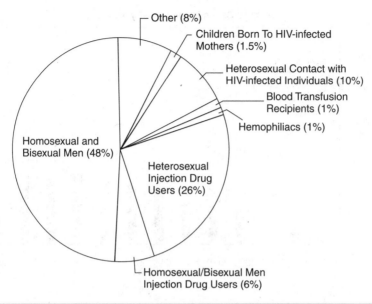

Other (8%)

Children Born To HIV-infected Mothers (1.5%)

Heterosexual Contact with HIV-infected Individuals (10%)

Blood Transfusion Recipients (1%)

Hemophiliacs (1%)

Homosexual and Bisexual Men (48%)

Heterosexual Injection Drug Users (26%)

Homosexual/Bisexual Men Injection Drug Users (6%)

Figure 6–2

Distribution of AIDS cases in the USA by risk group. (Cumulative figures, 1981–December, 1998)

ers. For a small percentage of cases (about 8 percent), no risk group has been assigned, perhaps because of the unavailability of information about the patients or their reluctance to acknowledge membership in a high-risk group. Women make up 16.5 percent of American AIDS cases; this low percentage is because the largest number of cases occur in homosexual and bisexual men. Women make up about half of the AIDS cases for the other risk groups.

Figure 6–3 shows the distribution of AIDS cases according to ethnicity. There is a disproportional number of AIDS cases among minorities, particularly African Americans and Hispanics. Indeed, although these groups make up about 23 percent of the general population, they make up 55 percent of AIDS cases—and an even higher percentage (80%) of the cases associated with in-jection drug use. Put another way, the frequency of AIDS cases among African Americans and Hispanics is about three to five times higher than in the general population. This points out the urgency of developing public health and educational measures targeted to these communities to control the epidemic.

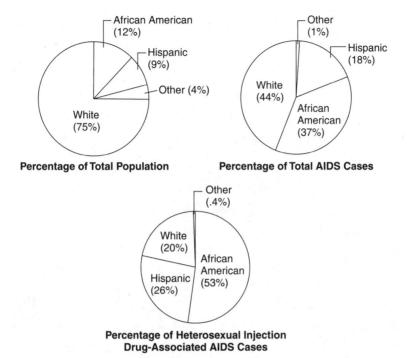

Percentage of Total Population

Percentage of Total AIDS Cases

Percentage of Heterosexual Injection Drug-Associated AIDS Cases

Figure 6–3

AIDS cases by ethnicity in the USA. (Cumulative figures, 1981–December, 1998)

The epidemiological data described in this section provide a current picture of HIV/AIDS in the United States. It is important to bear in mind that this picture can change as the AIDS epidemic progresses. This is addressed on page 130.

Epidemiology and Modes of HIV Transmission

Transmission of HIV is addressed in detail in Chapter 7. However, some examples of epidemiological studies regarding HIV transmission are presented here to illustrate how these studies allow us to draw conclusions about the relative risks of different activities for HIV transmission. One study implicates an activity (anal sex) in HIV transmission, and another study shows that casual contact does not cause HIV transmission. In addition, the possibility of HIV transmission by insects is considered.

Anal sex—a high-risk mode   Let's consider an epidemiological study that looked at the relative risks of different sexual activities. This study was part of the San Francisco Men's Health
Study, which is an ongoing cohort study of single men in an area
of that city. This particular area has been especially hard hit by
the AIDS epidemic. The study involved 1,034 single men, who
were monitored for HIV antibody status and asked about their
sexual practices. Of the homosexual men in this cohort, 48 percent were seropositive at the beginning. A low percentage (17.6
percent) of men who had refrained from sex during the previous
two years were seropositive, and this could be traced to sexual activity before that time. Table 6–2 shows frequencies of HIV infection when the homosexual men in the study were divided
according to whether or not they practiced anal intercourse.
Those who were the receptive partner or who were both receptive
and insertive showed significantly higher frequencies of HIV infection than those who did not engage in anal sex. This shows
that anal intercourse is a high-risk mode of HIV infection.

The results also showed that those who practiced only insertive anal intercourse were at less risk—in fact, this particular

Table 6–2
**HIV INFECTION IN HOMOSEXUAL MEN:
THE RELATIVE RISK OF ANAL SEX***

Sexual Practices for the Preceding Two Years	Percent HIV Seropositive (Adjusted for Number of Sexual Contacts)
No anal sex	20.6%
Anal sex, insertive only	26.7%
Anal sex, receptive only	44.6%
Anal sex, both insertive and receptive	53.3%

*These data are from the San Francisco Men's Study, as reported by Winkelstein
et al. (J. Amer. Med. Assoc. 257:321 [1987]). Individuals who did not practice
anal sex for the previous two years included those who practiced oral sex only
and also those who abstained entirely. The strongest correlation for HIV
seropositivity in this study was the number of sexual contacts an individual had.
The percentages in the table were adjusted to account for the average number of
sexual contacts for the different groups.

study could not statistically distinguish those men from men who did not engage in anal sex at all. However, other studies of heterosexual couples (who engage in vaginal as well as anal intercourse) clearly show that insertive intercourse can result in HIV transmission to the man. Thus, the most likely situation is that anal receptive intercourse is a very-high-risk sexual activity, and insertive intercourse is somewhat lower, although significant, in risk.

Casual contact—no measurable risk for HIV transmission
Casual contact with HIV-infected individuals poses no risk for infection. This was determined early in the epidemic, since people living with AIDS patients did not develop signs of HIV infection or AIDS. Casual contact includes hugging, touching, dry kissing, sharing of eating or drinking utensils, and sharing the workplace, telephones, and the like.

An example of an epidemiological study establishing that casual contact does not lead to HIV infection is shown in Table 6–3. One hundred and one individuals who shared a household with an AIDS patient for at least three months were tested for the presence of HIV antibodies. Only one person was seropositive, and this individual was a child of two injection drug users. Further investigation showed that this child acquired the infection at birth and not through casual contact. Thus, none of the individuals in this study became HIV infected through casual contact.

The results in Table 6–3 show that the risk of contracting HIV by casual contact is quite low, but this study could not rule out the possibility that casual contact could result in infrequent spread of HIV infection (because the number of subjects studied was not too large). However, in the more than ten years that have elapsed since this study was reported, no documented cases have been reported of HIV transmission by casual contact. Thus, it is safe to state that casual contact does not lead to transmission of HIV.

Insect bites—no evidence for spread of HIV   Early in the AIDS epidemic, some people claimed that insect bites could be a source of infection because insects such as mosquitoes draw a blood meal from the person they are biting, and they move from

Table 6–3
HIV INFECTION IN CASUAL HOUSEHOLD CONTACTS OF AIDS PATIENTS[1]

	Number Tested	Number HIV Seropositive
Children less than 6 years old	21	1[2]
Offspring of an AIDS patient	15	1[2]
Offspring of others	6	0
Children 6 to 18 years old	47	0
Adults	33	0
Total tested	101	

[1]The subjects in this study had lived in the same household with an AIDS patient for at least three months. Individuals who were in known high-risk groups (sexual relations with the AIDS patient, injection drug use, homosexual men) were not included. Thus, only individuals who had casual contact with the AIDS patient were studied. Among this group, 48 percent shared drinking glasses with the AIDS patient, 25 percent shared eating utensils, 9 percent shared razor blades, 90 percent shared toilets, and 37 percent shared beds. The AIDS patient was hugged by 79 percent of the subjects, kissed on the cheek by 83 percent, and kissed on the lips by 17 percent.

[2]Further investigation showed that the one seropositive child was the offspring of two injection drug abusers and probably acquired the infection at birth; this is a known mechanism of HIV transmission. Thus, none of these casual household contacts of AIDS patients became infected. These data are taken from a report by Friedland et al. (New England J. Med. 314:3244 [1986]).

person to person. However, epidemiological evidence argues against insect transmission of HIV. First of all, in well-studied North American or European populations, the great majority (about 97 percent) of AIDS cases can be explained by the well-documented modes of transmission. This includes a study in Belle Glade, Florida where some people proposed an outbreak of AIDS due to insect transmission. Furthermore, in Africa, where the insect populations are high, the age and geographical distributions of HIV infection argue against insect transmission. HIV is rare in children and the elderly, even in households where there are HIV-infected individuals. The old and the young are actually more frequently bitten by mosquitoes and other insects. In terms of geographical distribution, HIV infection is at high frequency in certain cities and urban areas, and there is much lower frequency of infection in surrounding rural areas. This is actually opposite from the pattern that would be expected if insects transmitted HIV, since they are more plentiful in rural areas.

Likelihood of Progression to AIDS

One very important concern is the likelihood of an HIV-infected individual eventually developing clinical AIDS. Prospective cohort studies have followed HIV-seropositive individuals for development of AIDS or ARC. An example of one study is shown in Table 6–4. After about four years of observation, 18 percent of the seropositive individuals developed AIDS, and an additional 47 percent developed signs of immunological impairment. Only 35 percent remained asymptomatic. Other similar studies currently predict that in the United States, most individuals infected with HIV (i.e., more than 70 percent) will develop AIDS or ARC within eight to ten years of infection if they do not receive antiviral therapy.

Table 6–4
LONG-TERM RESULTS OF HIV IN INFECTED MEN*

	Number of Individuals	Percent Total
AIDS	10	17.5
Signs of Immunological Damage		
LAS	16	28.1
Others (oral candidiasis, weight loss, etc.)	11	19.3
Subtotal	27	47.4
Asymptomatic	20	35.1

*Men in this study were followed for an average of 44 months after they showed initial signs of HIV infection (seroconversion). These data are taken from Ward et al. ("AIDS," G. P. Wormser et al., eds., Noyes Publications, Park Ridge, NJ [1987], pp 18–35).

This study was carried out before antiviral drugs were available. Today the development of AIDS would be much slower in individuals taking triple combination therapies.

The Effectiveness of AZT

As described in Chapter 4, p. 74, azidothymidine (AZT) was the first antiviral agent effective in AIDS. Previous laboratory experiments had shown that the drug could block HIV infection in isolated culture systems, and the drug was tested in a clinical trial, which can also be considered an interventional epidemiological study. Results from the first clinical trial of AZT are shown in Table 6–5. AIDS patients who had experienced one bout of *pneumocystis* pneumonia were divided into two groups. One group received AZT, and the other, control group received placebo pills that contained no drug. The physical states of all of the subjects were then monitored on a regular basis. After the study was in progress for less than six months, the results showed markedly better survival of the group taking AZT than the control group. In fact, the results were so striking that the investigators terminated the trial early and administered AZT to the control patients as well. Withholding the drug would have been unethical at that point. These studies led to approval of AZT for therapy in AIDS. Similar studies led to the approval of the other HIV antiviral drugs available today.

The Changing Face of AIDS

Earlier in this chapter we saw the epidemiological statistics for HIV and AIDS in the United States, in cumulative terms (Figures

Table 6–5
EFFECT OF AZIDOTHYMIDINE TREATMENT ON SURVIVAL OF AIDS PATIENTS*

Treatment	Number of Subjects	Number of Deaths	Percent Deaths
None (Placebo pills)	97	19	19.6
AZT	124	1	0.8

*The subjects were in the study an average of 16 to 17 weeks. The study was intended to last 24 weeks (6 months), but it was terminated early, once the dramatic effect of AZT treatment became evident. All subjects were offered AZT at that time. These data are taken from the report of the first large-scale test of AZT (Fishl et al., *New England J. Med.* 317:185 [1987]).

6–1, 6–2, and 6–3). It is important to remember that these statistics represent the cumulative experience with HIV infection since the beginning of the epidemic. However, the distribution of HIV infection in populations at risk changes with time; as HIV infection moves through different populations at different rates, the distribution of infection changes. Some examples are shown in Figures 6–4 and 6–5. From the beginning of the AIDS epidemic through 1986, homosexual and bisexual men made up 73 percent of the AIDS cases. By 1996 they represented 54 percent of the cumulative AIDS cases. This change represents the fact that relative to other risk groups, spread of HIV infection in homosexual and bisexual men during the 1980s and early 1990s increased more slowly. Likewise, in 1986, 60 percent of cumulative AIDS patients were white, but in 1996 only 46 percent were. This reflects the HIV/AIDS epidemic disproportionately affecting the Hispanic and African American communities in recent years.

The changes in AIDS distribution also make clear that current statistics on HIV/AIDS distributions do not tell us where HIV infection is spreading most rapidly. For instance, in the United States young adults are among the groups in which HIV infection is increasing most rapidly, although they do not currently make up the largest number of AIDS cases. Development of clinical AIDS takes several years, so individuals who become infected with HIV today may not impact the statistics for several years.

In the next section we will see that the worldwide distribution of HIV infection and AIDS cases is also changing rapidly.

AIDS AROUND THE WORLD

AIDS was first recognized as a disease in the United States. However, from the worldwide perspective, HIV infections in the United States and Western Europe represent a small fraction of the total cases. Estimates by public health officials are that in mid-1999, there were 34 million people in the world living with HIV infection and/or AIDS. From the beginning of the epidemic, nearly 47 million people have been infected by HIV. Approximately 95 percent of HIV-infected people are currently living in developing countries, with more than 90 percent living in sub-Saharan Africa

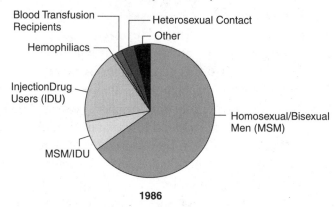

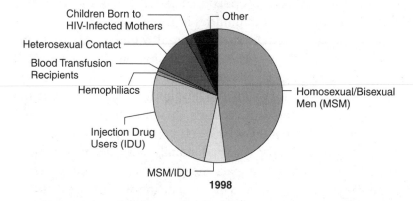

Figure 6–4

Cumulative AIDS cases by risk group are shown as of 1986, and as of 1998. These statistics represent the total cases since the beginning of the epidemic, and AIDS takes several years to develop. Therefore, the proportions of *new* HIV infections associated with homosexual/bisexual men may be even lower, and the proportions associated with heterosexual contact and injection drug use may be even higher. Homosexual and bisexual men are also referred to as men who have sex with men (MSM).

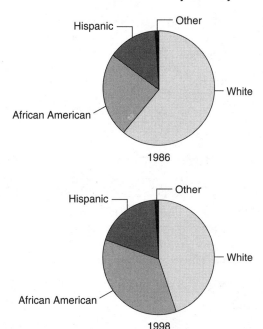

 Figure 6–5

Cumulative AIDS cases by ethnicity are shown as of 1986 and as of 1998. These represent the total cases since the beginning of the epidemic to those two dates.

or southern and Southeast Asia alone. The distribution of HIV infection throughout the world is illustrated in Figure 6–6.

It is important to consider control of HIV/AIDS in the global perspective for two reasons. First, HIV-infected people in all areas of the world develop the same immunodeficiency that is seen in developed countries, and the amount of suffering is equivalent. Second, it is in the self-interest of developed countries to combat infections such as HIV wherever they occur worldwide. In this age of rapid transportation, an infectious disease is only an airplane ride away from any place in the world. Thus, any HIV in the world is a threat to those of us in the United States. It is in our own self-interest to combat the spread of HIV on any continent.

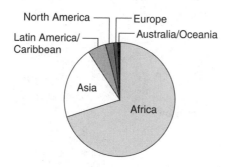

Worldwide Distribution of HIV Infection

Figure 6–6

The worldwide distribution of HIV infection. The distribution shown is taken from estimates by the MAP (Monitoring the AIDS Pandemic) Network, as of June 1998. These are estimates because reporting of HIV infection is incomplete in some parts of the world.

AIDS in Africa

AIDS is a major health problem in sub-Saharan Africa. The disease is centered in countries of central Africa, including the Democratic Republic of the Congo (Zaire), Kenya, Uganda, Zambia, Tanzania, and Rwanda. In contrast to the distribution of cases in North America and Europe, HIV infection is distributed more equally among men and women, and epidemiology shows that a predominant mode of transmission is heterosexual intercourse. Other modes of transmission may include blood transfusions, injections with reused needles, and procedures that involve scraping the skin with surgical knives (scarifications). The epidemic probably spread along truck routes through central Africa, and female prostitutes have been important reservoirs for the infection. The AIDS epidemic is mostly concentrated in cities and urban areas and is lower in rural areas. As in North America and Europe, the spread of HIV infection in Africa is a recent phenomenon, occurring mostly in the 1980s.

The extent of HIV infection in sub-Saharan Africa is alarmingly high. For example, as many as 90 percent of female prostitutes in Nairobi, Kenya, are HIV infected today. In 1985–1986, 18 percent of men visiting venereal disease clinics in Nairobi were seropositive for HIV, and the percentage has rapidly climbed since then. As many as 25 percent of the sexually active populations of some cities in Rwanda may be infected. In 1998, it was estimated that there were 24 million HIV-infected individuals in Africa, many of whom will probably progress to AIDS and eventually die. This will have devastating social and economic impact on these countries and may reach the proportions of some of the ancient epidemics described in Chapter 2.

The magnitude of the HIV/AIDS epidemic in Africa is compounded because these developing countries have limited financial abilities to provide medical care to HIV-infected patients. In particular, antiviral drugs (most notably the triple combination therapies), as well as drugs for many of the opportunistic infections, are beyond the reach of most HIV-infected patients in Africa. Thus, intervening in HIV transmission through preventive measures (and ultimately through the use of a vaccine) takes on even greater importance.

One factor that has increased the rates of HIV transmission in African populations is co-infection with sexually transmitted diseases (STDs) that cause sores in the genital tract tissues (for instance syphilis and chancroid). This makes sense because these infections allow the HIV virus or HIV-infected cells easier access to CD4 T-cells during sexual intercourse. Epidemiological studies have found that public health measures that decrease STD infections also decrease the rate of HIV transmission.

Another virus related to HIV has also been discovered in Africa. The original HIV that is associated with the great majority of AIDS cases is called *HIV-1* (see Chapter 4, p. 61). The other virus is called *HIV-2* and is predominantly found in countries along the west African coast, such as Senegal and the Ivory Coast. Molecular biological experiments tell us that HIV-1 and HIV-2 are closely related but distinct viruses that evolved from a common ancestor thousands of years ago. HIV-2 also causes AIDS, although there are some indications that it is less able to cause disease than HIV-1.

The existence of HIV-2 raises a problem since the standard HIV-1 ELISA tests do not detect HIV-2 antibodies. Thus, the standard HIV test will not detect individuals infected with HIV-2. So far in North America, few cases of HIV-2 infection have been found. However, it may be important to screen blood supplies and individuals for HIV-2 infection as well, to avoid undetected contamination or infections.

AIDS in Asia

While the largest number of HIV infections is currently in Africa, the world region where HIV infection is increasing most rapidly on a percentage basis is Asia. After HIV enters a high-risk population, it can spread extremely rapidly, if proper precautions (e.g., safer sex practices, injection drug precautions) are not taken. In the early 1980s, infection rates in most Asian countries were relatively low. However, HIV infection has begun to spread rapidly among commercial sex workers and injection drug users in India, Thailand, Myanmar (Burma), and Malaysia. In these countries, heterosexual sex and injection drug use are the major routes of infection. The levels of infection and the rates of increase in the high-risk populations are striking. For instance, in one six-month period (January to July 1988), the percentage of HIV-positive injection drug users monitored by one Bangkok hospital climbed from 1 percent to more than 30 percent. Fortunately, with the adoption of new public health measures in the mid-1990s, the rate of new infections in Thailand has begun to level off. In 1996, 36 percent of patients attending sexually transmitted disease clinics in Bombay (Mambai) were HIV positive and 50 percent of prostitutes were infected. It is estimated that there are 5 million infected people in India today, and that number is increasing unchecked. As in other parts of the world, the concern is that without intervention, these infections will spread into other populations in these countries, leading to the situations that confront many sub-Saharan African countries today. In fact, India now is the country with the largest number of HIV infections in the world, although several African countries have higher prevalence rates.

It is important to note that these figures represent HIV-infected individuals (detected by the antibody test described in Chapter 4, p. 68), not AIDS cases. Since most of these infected individuals acquired the virus relatively recently, most have not begun to show signs of illness yet. However, we can predict that within a few years, the number of AIDS cases in these countries will soar. Since there are not very many cases of full-blown AIDS in these countries yet, it is easy for the general public (and politicians) to ignore or downplay the problem for the time being.

There are differences between the HIV-1s that infect different parts of the world. These differences are largely in the envelope gene of the virus. The HIV-1s have been divided into subtypes or *clades;* there are now more than ten clades of HIV-1. In the United States and northern Europe, the predominant HIV-1 is clade B; in Africa, most of the HIV-1 clades are found; and in Asia, the predominant infections are by clade C and clade E viruses. The existence of different HIV-1 clades has two practical implications. First, distinguishing between different clades has allowed epidemiologists to more accurately track the spread of infection from one location to another. For instance, there are actually two HIV epidemics going on in Thailand: one epidemic involves heterosexual transmission in the northeastern part of the country (clade E HIV-1), and the other epidemic involving injection drug use is centered around Bangkok (clade B HIV-1). Second, the envelope proteins of the different HIV-1 clades are sufficiently different that some ELISA assay tests do not detect viruses of very different clades. Thus, diagnostic assays for HIV must be tailored to the virus infecting the community being tested. It has also been suggested that HIVs of different clades may differ somewhat in their ability to establish infection and/or cause disease.

The worldwide nature of HIV infection makes it a very important public health problem. No continents or countries are safe from infection, and the virus can spread rapidly (and undetected) once it enters a group engaging in high-risk behaviors.

In previous chapters, we analyzed how the AIDS virus operates at the cellular level and at the organism level. Now our focus shifts to the interorganism level. In this chapter, we look specifically at the question of how HIV is transmitted from person to person. Because there currently is no cure for AIDS once an individual has contracted the disease, preventing the transmission of HIV from person to person is critical. Consequently, in this chapter, we consider risk factors for HIV transmission and discuss ways of reducing these risk factors.

The evidence for assigning risks to different levels of activities comes from two main sources: theoretical biological considerations and empirical epidemiological data, bolstered by laboratory data. Theoretical analysis considers the biological plausibility of HIV transmission for particular activities based on the presence or absence of substances containing HIV and of receptors for these substances. For example, we know that HIV is not present in someone's exhaled breath; consequently, on the basis of theoretical analysis alone, we would assign little risk to breathing the air in the same room with a person with AIDS.

Theoretical analysis can be used to make predictions about no-, low-, or high-risk activities. These ultimately can be tested by empirical epidemiological data, the other main source of evidence for our risk judgments in this chapter. To continue the example above, epidemiological data from the sample of individuals who have lived with people with AIDS provide corroborating evidence that breathing the same air does not spread HIV (see Chapter 6, Table 6–3). Because epidemiological data indicate no AIDS incidence among family and friends who have simply lived with people with AIDS without intimate contact, and because of the biological implausibility, we can confidently state that breathing the same air is not a risk factor.

Typically, it is those activities with a high biological plausibility of HIV transmission that are carefully investigated with epidemiological studies. We saw one example of this in the last chapter. Anal receptive sexual activity has a high biological plausibility of HIV transmission, and the evidence from epidemiological studies discussed in Chapter 6 (Table 6–2) provides corroborative evidence that this behavior is, in fact, strongly associated with HIV infection.

In addition, epidemiological evidence can provide the initial evidence that certain activities are or are not associated with HIV infection risk. At the outset of the AIDS epidemic, for instance, it was epidemiological studies that led to the identification of likely modes of HIV transmission. This, in part, guided subsequent biological laboratory work, aided in the theoretical understanding of AIDS, and resulted in the isolation of HIV.

We should remember one aspect of epidemiological information at the outset of our discussion of risk and risk factors. Epidemiological studies have identified certain groups of individuals who are overrepresented in the population of those with AIDS: in particular, gay and bisexual men and injection drug users make up a large percentage of those with AIDS. There is nothing about being gay, bisexual, or an injection drug user that, by itself, leads to HIV infection and AIDS. Rather, individuals in these groups are, on average, more likely to undertake certain *behaviors* that have a high biological plausibility of HIV transmission. Because of these higher HIV-risk behaviors among some people in the group, the likelihood of transmission averaged over the whole group increases, if the necessary and sufficient behaviors for HIV transmission occur.

Consider, for example, two cases: a homosexual man (Jim) who has unprotected anal sex with another homosexual man, and a heterosexual woman (Susan) who has unprotected vaginal sex with a heterosexual man. Assume that neither Jim nor Susan is HIV positive. In each case, Jim and Susan are involved in behaviors that have a high biological plausibility for HIV transmission. The important and unknown factor, then, is the HIV status of their partners. On the sole basis of average U.S. HIV infection rates, which are higher among gay men as a group than among heterosexual men as a group, Jim is at more risk than Susan. However, without complete data on their partners' HIV status and sexual history, neither Jim nor Susan can be certain of their risk for this particular sexual encounter. The safest approach, as we shall see below, is to avoid unprotected anal or vaginal intercourse.

Before we consider the risks of particular behaviors, however, we need to understand the biological bases of HIV transmission, including such issues as the primary sources of HIV within an infected person, the stability of the virus in moving between individuals, and the targets for infection in an uninfected individual.

BIOLOGICAL BASES OF HIV TRANSMISSION

In infected people, infectious HIV is present only in cells and some human body fluids. Despite its devastating effects within the body, the virus is actually quite fragile in the external environment and dies quickly when exposed to room temperature and air conditions. In fact, very special laboratory conditions are needed to grow HIV outside the human body. It is important to remember this fact because it is easy to assume—mistakenly—that a disease as deadly as AIDS must be caused by an agent that is tremendously strong and sturdy. People's fears of the disease, combined with their lack of knowledge and mistaken impressions about epidemics, can cause them to view HIV in an anthropomorphic way—almost like a living, breathing enemy capable of thought and devastating action. Instead, the reality of HIV outside the body is much different: a fragile virus that loses infectivity quickly.

Sources of Infectious HIV

In an infected individual, HIV is present in certain cells, as well as in some bodily fluids and secretions, many of which also contain these cells. In terms of cells, macrophages and T_{helper} lymphocytes are susceptible to infection by HIV, as described in Chapter 4. Macrophages may be the long-term reservoirs of HIV in infected individuals because they are not killed by the virus. Macrophages circulate through the bloodstream, and they also are found in all mucosal linings of the body, such as the internal urogenital surface of the vagina and penis and the lining of the anus, lungs, and throat. Another kind of cell that can be infected with HIV is the

Langerhans cell, found on mucosal surfaces and below the surface of the skin.

Among people who test positive for HIV, the virus is not found consistently in all body fluids and products. Furthermore, in body fluids where HIV is regularly found, it occurs in different concentrations at different times. Nonetheless, we can place the body fluids and products into three groups based on the degree of association between body fluids/products and HIV infection. These groupings reflect differences among body fluids/products in their general concentrations of infectious HIV or HIV-infected cells and in the amount of relative exposure a typical individual might experience. Table 7–1 lists these groupings.

Researchers have developed methods to test for HIV and estimate the amounts of infectious virus present in various body fluids and secretions. HIV can be isolated relatively easily from blood, semen, and vaginal/cervical secretions (including menstrual fluid). When blood and semen are examined closely, the great majority of HIV is associated with infected cells (mostly macrophages) present in these fluids. In blood, if the cells are removed, low levels of HIV are present in the cell-free serum. It has also been isolated from breast milk. With much greater difficulty, the virus has, on occasion, been isolated from saliva, tears, and

Table 7–1
DEGREE OF ASSOCIATION BETWEEN HIV INFECTION AND DIFFERENT BODY FLUIDS AND PRODUCTS

Group 1: Very High Association*

Blood	Semen	Vaginal/Cervical Secretion (incl. menstrual fluid)

Group 2: High Association

Breast Milk

Group 3: Low or No Association

Saliva	Tears	Perspiration/Sweat
Urine	Feces	

*The amount of infectious HIV in these fluids is particularly high in individuals during the initial (acute) phase of infection and in individuals with clinical AIDS.

urine. It has not been isolated from perspiration and feces. The current scientific view is that body fluids and products other than blood, semen, vaginal/cervical secretions, and breast milk contain so little, if any, HIV that they are not of major importance in HIV transmission between individuals.

Blood, semen, and vaginal/cervical secretions are of greatest concern when we consider HIV transmission due to another factor: These are the most infectious fluids to which a potential target individual might be exposed during activities typically associated with HIV transmission (sexual behavior or injection drug use). These issues are covered in detail later in this chapter. The relative HIV infectivity of different body fluids and products can be explained in another way, using biological considerations.

The fluids and products listed in Table 7–1 differ in the amount of live cells they contain. Blood, semen, vaginal/cervical secretions, and breast milk contain high numbers of live cells. The other body fluids and products (saliva, tears, perspiration, urine, and feces) are completely or nearly completely free of live cells (although they may contain nonhuman cells, such as bacteria). Because live infected cells produce HIV, we would expect fluids with live cells to pose the greatest risks for HIV transmission.

Stability of HIV

For transmission of HIV infection to occur, infectious virus must survive long enough to pass to a susceptible person and infect target cells. The HIV virus particle (see Chapter 4) is actually a very fragile one, as discussed earlier. As a result, the virus quickly becomes inactivated when exposed to the drying effects of air or light. It is also quickly inactivated by contact with soap and water.

As mentioned, much of the infectious HIV is associated with cells (macrophages and T-lymphocytes). In blood or semen, cells maintain infectious HIV as long as they themselves are alive. Thus, intravenous transfusions or sexual intercourse involving HIV-infected individuals efficiently transmits infection, since live cells are passed. On the other hand, if blood or semen is allowed to dry, the cells die quickly and the HIV infectivity is lost.

These facts about the stability of HIV, combined with the facts about likely sources of HIV infection, explain why casual contact with people with AIDS does not result in the spread of HIV infection (see Chapter 6 and below).

Targets for HIV Infection

At the cellular level, HIV infection requires the presence of virus receptors on the cell surface. As described in Chapter 4, the receptor for HIV is the CD4 surface protein, which is present only on T_{helper} lymphocytes, macrophages, and the Langerhans cells. Thus, these are the cells that become infected in a susceptible individual. These cells are most abundant in the blood. Consequently, activities that introduce infectious HIV, either as infected cells or free virus, into the blood of an uninfected individual has the potential to result in infection. For example, sexual intercourse can result in damage or (sometimes microscopic) tears of the mucosal linings of the female genital tracts or of the male or female rectum. These tears can allow passage of blood or semen into the circulatory system of the uninfected individual. In addition, as described above, macrophages and Langerhans cells are also present at the mucosal surfaces of the rectum and genital tract, and they potentially can be infected directly without the necessity of virus entry into the bloodstream.

Other potential targets for HIV infection are the oral cavity and the throat. Like the genital tract and the rectum, the throat's mucosal lining contains macrophages and Langerhans cells. In certain sexual activities, such as oral sex, semen can be exchanged orally from one person to another. Consequently, there is the theoretical potential for infection. The epidemiological reality, however, is that oral sex is not a primary mode of transmission of HIV, as we shall see later. The explanation for this may be that there is less physical trauma associated with oral sex or that chemical and physiological features of the oral cavity reduce the efficiency of transmission. This case demonstrates the need to combine theoretical predictions from biology with epidemiological data about incidence rates to understand fully the risks of HIV transmission. It is this topic to which we now turn.

Modes of HIV Transmission

We are now ready to analyze the modes of HIV transmission from person to person and the relative risks associated with different modes. In making our assessment of risk, we will rely on both the plausibility of HIV transmission, based on theoretical biological analysis, and the empirical facts associating documented HIV transmission with various modes, drawn from epidemiological studies. Together, these two sources of information permit us to categorize activities and behaviors according to the degree of their association with HIV infection.

No Association with HIV Transmission: Casual Contact

Because HIV is so fragile outside the body, transmission requires direct contact of two substances: fluid containing infectious HIV from an infected person and susceptible cells (usually via the bloodstream) of another person. Because of the absence of this type of direct contact, a large group of interpersonal activities and behaviors, generally referred to as casual contact, have no measured association with HIV transmission (see Chapter 6, p. 127) and therefore pose no risk for HIV infection.

What do we mean by *casual contact*? This includes all types of ordinary, everyday, nonsexual contacts between and among people. Shaking hands, hugging, kissing, sharing eating utensils, sharing towels or napkins, using the same telephone, and using the same toilet seat are a few examples of casual contact. It is impossible to list all types of casual contact here, but we can analyze or make predictions about others, keeping in mind the need for direct contact with body fluids containing infectious HIV. For example, consider the possibilities of waterborne or airborne transmission. Because HIV is quickly inactivated outside the body, it cannot survive in the open air or in water. Consequently, we would predict that there is no risk in sharing the same physical space with a person with AIDS or swimming in the same pool. Epidemiological evidence supports this conclusion: There is no measured risk of transmission.

Activities Associated with HIV Transmission

HIV transmission occurs when there is direct contact between HIV-tainted fluid from an infected person and the bloodstream or a mucosal lining of another person. Epidemiological data point to three modes of HIV transmission from person to person: via birth, via blood, or via sex. For most people, the last mode of transmission—via sex—is the most likely, and we discuss it at length later. First, however, we will briefly discuss the other two modes. These are listed in Table 7–2 and discussed below.

Perinatal Transmission from an Infected Mother to Her Gestating Infant

This mode of HIV transmission brings together a source of HIV (in the bloodstream of an HIV-infected woman) and a potential target (the bloodstream of a developing fetus) in a protected environment (the mother's womb). The mother's and child's bloodstreams are separated by the placenta, which prevents exchange of cells but not of nutrients. During the third trimester of pregnancy, however, small tears sometimes occur in the placenta, which can lead to entry of cells from the mother's bloodstream into the child's. In addition, during birth, the child frequently comes into close contact with or swallows the mother's cervical-vaginal secretions or blood due to the bleeding normally associated with delivery. Although reports vary, a good estimate is that there is about a 23 percent chance that a child of an infected mother will be infected if there is no antiviral treatment (see Chapter 5, p. 105). Intensive treatment, however, of the mother during pregnancy and delivery and of the infant during the first six weeks of life can reduce the transmission rate to 8 percent.

Table 7–2
MODES OF HIV TRANSMISSION

1. Birth: Perinatal transmission from an infected mother to her gestating infant.
2. Blood: Transmission from an HIV-infected source to the bloodstream.
3. Sex: Intimate sexual contact with an HIV-infected person.

Transmission from an HIV-Infected Source to the Bloodstream

This mode of transmission relates to receiving blood or blood products. This can occur in two main ways: by receiving a transfusion of HIV-infected blood or by injection with an HIV-contaminated syringe (either accidentally or incidentally).

Receiving a transfusion of HIV-infected blood. Since a transfusion involves placing foreign blood or blood products directly into the recipient's bloodstream, the necessary conditions for HIV transmission are present: direct contact of potentially infected fluid with susceptible cells in the recipient. Before 1985, when screening of the blood supply for HIV by the antibody test was begun (see Chapter 4, p. 68), the sufficient condition for contracting AIDS was present: HIV-infected blood for transfusion. Even then, however, the risk was low that the blood or blood product involved in a transfusion was infected—except for hemophiliacs who required a clotting factor extracted from the blood of many different donors. Now, this sufficient condition is very unlikely.

It is estimated that 18 million units of blood components are transfused per year in the United States. In 1984, the year before antibody test screening of the blood supply was begun, the risk of receiving HIV-infected blood was 40 out of 100,000. Now, the risk is 2.25 out of 100,000 (although one set of researchers believes the risk is even lower, at about half this rate). Why is there still some risk? This occurs because the screening tests are not perfect and because of the possibility that detectable antibodies have not yet developed in a recently infected donor. Compared with the risk of dying from a condition serious enough to require hospitalization and a blood transfusion (that is, 40 out of 100, or 40,000 out of 100,000, if the transfusion is refused), the risk of receiving HIV-infected blood during a transfusion is about 15,500 times less.

Blood donation centers have developed methods to reduce the risk even further (Fig. 7–1). In addition to routine screening using the tests discussed in Chapter 4, p. 68, centers have developed information campaigns that discourage blood donation from those who might be infected. New procedures also have been established to permit donors, particularly those who may feel pressured during a work-associated blood drive, to indicate

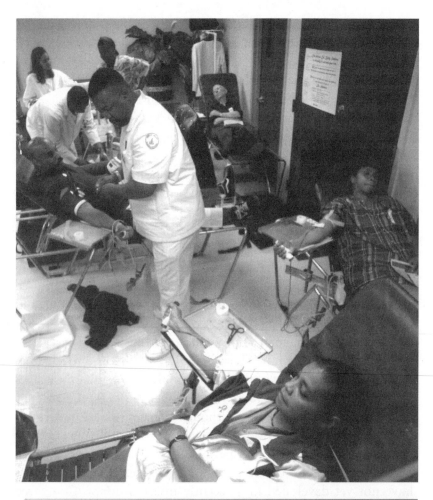

Figure 7-1

A blood donor center.

confidentially that their blood should not be used. The American Red Cross blood donation offices give all blood donors a special card describing a procedure that must be followed by all potential donors. The card lists nine groups of people who should not give blood, then describes a confidential procedure that all donors must follow, involving bar-code labels indicating "transfuse" or "do not transfuse." People in one of the nine groups (e.g., drug users, men who have had sex with men since 1977) are to remove the "do not transfuse" bar code tag and place it on another card.

Those not in one of the listed groups remove the "transfuse" bar code tag and place it on the card. The bar code tags are identical to the casual observer, but not to the optical scanner, which later identifies the blood to be rejected. As these procedures become routinely accepted by staff and donors, the risk of receiving infected blood or blood products from a transfusion will become even smaller.

Before we conclude this section, it is important to note two points. First, we have been analyzing the potential risks of receiving a blood transfusion, not of donating blood. There are no risks of HIV transmission from donating blood. The donor's blood is the only potential source of HIV in this situation: If there is no HIV in that blood, there is no other source of the virus. Second, receipt of an organ transplant is a possible source of HIV, were the organ donor HIV-infected. Like blood donations, organ donations are tested for HIV, so the risk is quite small. Sperm donations also could be HIV-infected and are screened for HIV.

Injecting oneself with HIV-infected blood. There are two ways in which HIV-contaminated blood in needles can lead to transmission: when needles are shared during injection drug use and through accidental needle sticks between HIV-infected individuals and health workers.

In the case of injection drug use, the two necessary elements are present: contaminated blood and direct injection of that blood into the bloodstream. During the process of injecting the drug, an individual draws blood into the syringe to be sure that the needle is in a vein. Infected blood, then, can be mixed with the drug solution. If the syringe is passed to another individual and inserted into his or her body, contaminated blood from the previous person can be passed into the bloodstream as part of the drug solution.

At first, this mode of transmission may appear contradictory, in that HIV is taken outside the body first, then passed to another individual. This occurs, however, in the special context of a protective container—the closed container of the syringe—where blood cells and virus are not exposed to the environment. In addition, it is generally done in a very short time, usually within seconds or, at most, minutes. Consequently, the blood cells remain alive and, with them, the HIV.

Prevention of this mode of transmission involves breaking the link between individuals via the syringe. Injection drug users are encouraged first not to share needles. Some cities provide free sterile needles so that limited syringe availability is not an issue. Alternatively, injection drug users are encouraged to clean their needles between administrations, using a bleach solution.

The other mode of HIV infection is via accidental needle sticks by health workers. On occasion, health workers, in emergencies or in the process of medical laboratory work with HIV-infected people, have accidentally stuck themselves with potentially contaminated needles. There are a total of about 800,000 needle sticks in the U.S. every year from syringes, various intravenous needle assemblies, and blood-draw equipment; of these, about 16,000, or 2 percent, are with HIV-contaminated devices. The risk of contracting HIV from a contaminated needle stick is about 1 in 200 (or one-half of one percent). Consequently, the risk that a health care worker will accidentally stick himself or herself with an HIV-contaminated needle and then develop HIV is 0.0001 percent. To put these figures in a larger perspective, it is instructive to compare the transmission rates of HIV and the hepatitis B virus (a virus transmitted by similar routes as HIV) by needle stick injuries. The rate for transmission of HIV via a contaminated needle stick is approximately 0.5 percent. In contrast, the rate of transmission for hepatitis B virus via a contaminated needle stick is between 6 and 30 percent.

The greatest risk of HIV infection for health care workers is by an accidental needle stick. As the data presented above show, however, this risk is, in fact, quite low. Nonetheless, the risk does exist, as does the relatively greater risk of contracting other infectious diseases such as hepatitis via needle sticks. Consequently, during clinical procedures, health workers (who also should be wearing gloves) have been advised to discard used needles directly rather than recap before discarding. In addition, new needles have been designed that make accidental sticks more difficult.

Intimate Sexual Contact with an HIV-Infected Person

For most people in the general public, this mode of transmission is the most likely source of HIV infection. The risk differs, however, depending on the particular sexual practice, the frequency of the practice, and the HIV status of a sexual partner. We cannot, therefore, categorize particular sexual practices with certainty in terms of their HIV risk. The degree of risk of any particular sexual behavior differs from person to person. Individual risk assessment, however, is usually a difficult task, based on incomplete and sometimes unknowable data (e.g., the HIV status of a new sexual partner).

To make this task somewhat easier, we can discuss what we know from the theoretical and epidemiological perspectives. Together, the data from these perspectives complement each other and provide useful information for judging the relative risk of various sexual practices.

From the theoretical perspective, we know that we need two critical elements together: HIV-contaminated body fluid (in particular, blood, semen, or cervical-vaginal secretions) and direct contact of this fluid with a target site. The riskiest sexual practices, therefore, are those in which HIV-infected blood, semen, or cervical-vaginal secretions from an infected person come in immediate and direct contact with the bloodstream or mucous membranes of another person. These practices include vaginal intercourse between a man and a woman, anal intercourse between a man and a woman, and anal intercourse between two men. In all of these practices, semen from the man is deposited into vagina or rectum—both sites of macrophages and Langerhans cells and also sites where small tears frequently occur during intercourse.

At the other end of the spectrum, the least risky sexual practices are those where HIV-infected blood, semen, or cervical-vaginal secretions do not usually come into contact with target sites. These practices include masturbation by a male onto unbroken skin of a partner and dry kissing (closed-mouth kissing). In the case of male masturbation, while potentially infected semen is present, a target site is not—unbroken skin of a partner. In the case of dry kissing, neither blood nor semen is usually present, and saliva of HIV-infected people has been shown to contain little or no HIV.

On this spectrum of risk, we can anchor the ends of potentially risky sexual behaviors but cannot precisely anchor other groups of sexual practices or consider every possible case that could arise. For example, what if two people are dry kissing and one has a cut on the lip: Is there a risk of HIV infection? Or, what if a man masturbates onto chapped skin: Is there a risk of HIV infection? The answer to both questions is "possibly." Here is where the epidemiological evidence is useful.

We know that, across groups of people, those who frequently engage in particular sexual practices are more likely to become HIV infected. The sexual practices listed above at the "riskiest" end of the spectrum of risk (vaginal intercourse with an HIV-infected person without a condom, anal intercourse with an HIV-infected person without a condom) have been shown, through epidemiological data, to be highly associated with HIV infection. The two practices from the "least-risky" end of the spectrum (dry kissing and masturbation by an HIV-infected male onto the unbroken skin of a partner) have not been shown, through epidemiological data, to be associated with HIV infection.

Epidemiological data also provide clues to the relative infectivity of other sexual practices. Wet kissing (open-mouth kissing with exchange of saliva) has not been shown to be associated with HIV transmission. This makes sense from a biological perspective too, since we know that saliva of an HIV-infected person contains little, if any, HIV. Oral sex performed on an HIV-infected man or woman by either a woman or a man has not been strongly associated with HIV transmission, although there are some reported cases of transmission via this sexual practice. From a biological perspective, we can see why this might be the case, if the HIV-infected semen is deposited in the mouth and throat or possibly into the bloodstream via small tears in the mouth. Still, there must be other chemical or physiological factors (e.g., the acidity of the mouth) that provide some barrier to HIV transmission because the epidemiological data do not show oral sex to be highly associated with HIV transmission.

From our analysis of the relative risk of various sexual practices based on biological and epidemiological considerations, we can not only place the sexual practices on the spectrum of HIV risk but also see ways to reduce the risks of all sexual practices that could involve some risk. Abstinence from sexual relations clearly reduces the risk of transmission to zero: no source and no target. Abstinence, however, is not an option that many sexually active people choose. These people can decide to have sexual relations of the least risky types. If they choose riskier sexual practices, they can reduce the risks by placing barriers between potential sources of HIV infection and potential targets. For example, they can use condoms during vaginal and anal intercourse to reduce the risk of HIV infection by containing potentially infected semen within the condom and preventing its contact with target sites in the vagina or rectum. Condom use during oral sex on a man also provides a barrier between potentially infectious semen and the target sites in the mouth and throat. During oral sex on a woman, a dental dam (a 3- to 4-inch square piece of latex) placed over the vagina also provides a barrier for source-to-target-site contact.

These protective methods are not 100 percent effective. Condoms can have holes and can leak; however, this is not at all frequent. Studies are regularly done on condom reliability, and condom manufacturers pay close attention to quality control procedures. Properly used, condoms provide a good measure of protection for most people. A condom should be fresh and made of latex (not of natural products). The condom must be placed on the man's erect penis prior to any penetration, since pre-ejaculatory fluid has been shown to be HIV infected in an HIV-infected individual. Space should be left in the tip of the condom for the semen that will soon be ejaculated, and the condom should be unrolled completely to the base of the erect penis. If a lubricant is used during intercourse, it should be water based, not grease or oil based, which destroys latex. Condoms or lubricants with nonoxynol-9, a spermicide, used to be recommended; recent studies, however, indicate that nonoxynol-9 does not kill the virus and may even cause irritation that could make HIV entry more likely. Consequently, condoms without nonoxynol-9 but with a water-based lubricant are now recommended. The condom must stay in place at the base of the penis until the penis is withdrawn from the vagina or rectum; this is best done before the man's erection fades and the penis is flaccid and separated from the stretched condom.

Each person has to analyze his or her own sexual practices and take the precautions necessary for protection from HIV. The guidelines described above for self-protection are similar to those advocated by the U.S. Surgeon General, the U.S. Centers for Disease Control, and many local AIDS prevention programs. The final decisions about individual risk assessment and management are made differently by each of us. Although we will never have all the data we need to make perfect decisions, we can make use of information from biological and epidemiological studies to assess the risks of various sexual practices. These assessments are best made before sexual activity, when our thinking is less affected by volatile emotions and judgment-confusing substances (alcohol or drugs), which are sometimes associated with sexual behavior for some people. Because sexual activity usually involves two people, it is necessary to think about HIV risk assessment and make decisions on HIV risk management together with your sexual partner before sexual activity. Then, those who choose to have sexual relations will be ready to enjoy the sexual experience more, knowing that they have taken the necessary precautions to lower the risk of HIV transmission.

CHAPTER 8
Future Directions in Combating AIDS

In this book, we have learned about AIDS in terms of basic biomedical aspects. We have considered the virus (HIV), the immune system, the physical manifestations of AIDS, and transmission of the virus. The fact remains that HIV infection is continuing to spread in many areas of the world, and there is currently no cure for the disease. How can we respond to this disease, and in what areas are we likely to see activity and progress?

FUTURE DIRECTIONS FOR BIOMEDICAL EFFORTS

The biomedical community will focus on two major problems regarding AIDS: (1) *prevention of infection through vaccines* and (2) *treatment of infected individuals who develop symptoms of the disease*. Let's look at some of the areas where current and future efforts are likely to focus.

Prevention of Infection

Research

Remarkable progress has been made in terms of biomedical research on AIDS in finding and studying the virus itself. Currently, the lack of a convenient animal model system is a major stumbling block. Faster progress could be made in understanding the disease process and testing vaccines and therapies if HIV caused a similar disease in experimental animals. However, HIV infects only man and higher apes, such as chimpanzees; furthermore, the virus does not readily cause disease in chimpanzees. Several retroviruses similar to HIV have been found in monkeys (SIVs, Chapter 4, p. 78), and one strain induces immunodeficiency in rhesus monkeys, so this has been a useful model system. However, monkeys are very expensive to maintain in laboratories, they are in short supply, and the use of primates in research is strongly opposed by some animal welfare advocates. Thus, other more convenient animal model systems are desirable. One possibility is cats: Two retroviruses of cats cause immunodeficiencies. One of these cat viruses (FIV) is a lentivirus.

Recently, it has been possible to grow cells of the human immune system in special mice. These mice carry a genetic defect called *severe combined immunodeficiency (SCID)*, which leaves them with crippled immune systems—much like those in AIDS patients. Because SCID mice lack functional cellular immunity, it is possible to implant them with human cells without tissue rejection taking place. Researchers have developed techniques to implant human fetal tissues containing stem cells for the blood into SCID mice. It is then possible to reconstitute these mice with functional human immune cells, including T-lymphocytes and B-lymphocytes. They have also found that if these SCID mice are infected by HIV, the virus will establish infection in the human tissue and destroy the T_{helper} lymphocytes, just as it does in humans. Thus, some of the mechanisms by which HIV attacks the immune system can be studied in these mice. In addition, they may be useful for testing potential antiviral drugs.

Another recent development has been production of hybrid *simian-human immunodeficiency viruses (SHIVs)* by gene cloning techniques. Since SIVs and HIVs are closely related, substitution of HIV genes into SIV often results in a hybrid virus that can still replicate. In particular, SHIVs that consist of the HIV-1 envelope gene inserted in place of an SIV can both replicate and cause AIDS in monkeys. These viruses are useful for studying the host immune response to HIV envelope protein during disease development. This kind of SHIV may be valuable for developing and testing anti-HIV vaccines. Other SHIVs may also be useful. For instance, an SHIV containing the HIV reverse transcriptase might be used to test the effectiveness in monkeys of antiviral drugs targeted at HIV reverse transcriptase.

Vaccines

Ideally, the most effective prevention of HIV infection would be a vaccine that blocks virus infection in an individual. Indeed, effective vaccines have been developed against most human viruses that cause serious diseases (for instance, smallpox, polio, measles, and influenza). Although several possible vaccines against HIV are under development, there are some theoretical reasons that it may be difficult to develop an effective one. As discussed in Chapter 4, p. 72, HIV evades the immune system in an infected individual. Briefly, this results from (1) the high mutation rate of the virus, particularly in the *env* gene; (2) the ability of the virus to establish a latent state in some cells; and (3) the ability of the virus to spread by cell-to-cell contact. The objective of a vaccine is to raise a protective immune response to the infectious agent. Since HIV evades the immune system so efficiently, it may be difficult for a vaccine to prevent HIV infection in an individual even if it can induce production of neutralizing antibodies or cell-mediated immunity. Another challenge for HIV vaccines is the differences between HIVs found in various parts of the world (see Chapter 6, p. 136). It will probably be necessary to tailor HIV vaccines to the targeted geographical areas.

Despite these theoretical concerns, a number of HIV vaccines have been under development. Most of them have been developed by state-of-the-art gene splicing (or recombinant DNA) techniques that have allowed large-scale production of individual viral proteins. The predominant HIV proteins that make up these potential vaccines are *env* proteins (e.g., gp120) and, to a lesser extent, *gag* proteins. In addition, inactivated whole HIV virus is being tested. Most of these vaccines can raise anti-HIV antibody responses when injected into monkeys or humans. A United States government–sponsored vaccine trial in humans was planned, but it was placed on hold because it was found that the test vaccines could not stimulate protection against HIV isolated directly from patients, although they could protect against HIV grown in the laboratory.

Considerable HIV vaccine research has focused on simian immunodeficiency viruses (SIVs) since they are closely related to HIV, and some SIV strains cause AIDS in certain monkey species. As mentioned earlier, chimpanzees are the only monkeys that HIV can infect, but the virus does not readily cause AIDS in these animals. Thus, many principles of HIV vaccines are being studied by developing analogous vaccines for SIV and testing their abilities to inhibit both SIV infection and disease in monkeys. A vaccine consisting of killed SIV virus particles has also been prepared. When this killed virus was used to immunize monkeys, it prevented them from developing viral infection or immunodeficiency when injected with low doses of live SIV virus. This was encouraging, but this vaccine protected only against low virus doses. Moreover, it could not protect from infection if live SIV-infected cells were injected—a situation probably closer to natural routes of HIV infection.

More recent experiments with the SIV model system raise the prospects for an attenuated live virus vaccine—analogous to the live poliovirus vaccine (Sabin vaccine) commonly used today. Researchers inactivated one of the SIV accessory genes (*nef*; see Chapter 4, p. 63), and they showed that this mutant SIV could still infect monkeys, but it does not induce disease. Moreover, prior infection with the *nef*-mutant SIV could efficiently protect monkeys from infection by normal SIV, and these monkeys did not develop immunodeficiency. The immunity induced by *nef*-mutant SIV was much stronger than that induced by the killed virus vaccine. HIV has a *nef* gene as well, which raises the possibility of generating a live, attenuated *nef*-mutant HIV as a vaccine. In this case, safety of an attenuated HIV vaccine in not inducing AIDS will be very important.

As we discussed in Chapter 3, there are two branches of the immune system: the humoral immune system produces antibody molecules, and the cellular immune system produces antigen-specific T-lymphocytes. Due to intricacies of the immune system, most of the anti-HIV vaccines originally tested were likely to induce anti-HIV antibody responses. However, if cellular immunity to HIV is important for resistance to HIV infection, these vaccines may not be effective. Vaccines designed to induce cellular immunity to HIV are under development as well. Several large-scale trials under way use combinations of vaccines designed to induce cellular immunity with ones that induce humoral immunity.

In all cases, the first steps for vaccine trials will simply determine if individuals injected with the test vaccines produce antibodies (or other immune responses) against HIV and if they experience no other harmful side effects (Phase I clinical trials; see below). In the initial trials, the proper doses of vaccine to produce an immune response are also determined. Once this has been established, then other, large-scale trials will test whether the vaccines are effective in preventing HIV infection. Some of the vaccines are currently moving through the vital clinical trial phases.

Testing an HIV vaccine in humans brings together scientific and societal issues. Because of the bioethical issues involved in using humans, groups of specialists in both the biomedical and psychological aspects of HIV and AIDS are working together to implement trials that take scientific, human, and societal considerations into account.

Treatment of Infected Individuals

Biomedical efforts to treat HIV-infected individuals will focus on three main areas: (1) *antivirals* that interfere with continued HIV infection, (2) *restoration of the immune system*, and (3) *treatments of opportunistic infections and cancers*.

Antivirals

As described in Chapters 4 and 5, several antiviral compounds are now approved for use in treatment of HIV-infected individuals and AIDS patients. These drugs are targeted against two of the HIV proteins: *reverse transcriptase* (nucleoside analogs such as AZT, and also non-nucleoside reverse transcriptase inhibitors), and *protease* (protease inhibitors). The fact that these drugs work means that agents that interfere with continued HIV infection in an AIDS patient will improve the clinical status. Thus, continued efforts are needed to develop new antiviral compounds that also block HIV infection. This is particularly important, since drug-resistant HIV frequently appears in infected individuals who are taking an antiviral drug (see Chapter 5, p. 103).

So far, all of the approved anti-HIV drugs work by interfering with processes carried out by the two viral enzymes reverse transcriptase and protease. Other potential antivirals could attack other "Achilles' heels" of the virus—processes that are vital to the virus but are not necessary for the survival of the host cell. Nine different genes carried by HIV specify proteins necessary for the virus's life cycle (Chapter 4). Any of these viral proteins are potential targets for new antiviral drugs. Some of the next targets for antiviral drug development will be the integrase enzyme (necessary for integration of viral DNA into the host cell's DNA) and the *tat* and *rev* regulatory proteins. Laboratory experiments have shown that if any of the genes for these viral proteins are disabled, then HIV cannot replicate. Thus, antiviral drugs that inhibit their function should also be effective at inhibiting HIV infection in people. So far, compounds have been identified that can inhibit the function of each of these viral proteins during HIV infection in laboratory cultures. Thus, these are potential new antiviral drugs, although none are near the stage where they might be approved for use.

Many additional steps lie between identification of a potential antiviral compound and establishing it as an effective and approved drug. Some of the questions that must be addressed during development of a drug are:

1. What methods are required to deliver effective doses of the compound into individuals?
2. Are there side effects *(toxicity)*, and can effective doses be delivered without side effects?
3. Does the compound actually inhibit HIV replication in humans?
4. Is the compound as effective or more effective than the currently available drugs?

Satisfying these questions takes an enormous amount of effort on the part of biomedical researchers, as well as a great deal of time. Development of a single antiviral drug requires many millions of dollars and typically five to ten years. In fact, many compounds that show antiviral activity in the laboratory ultimately will never be usable as an anti-HIV drug. Nevertheless, in some cases, a compound that shows some antiviral activity in the laboratory might be modified by pharmaceutical chemists into a compound with potency in HIV-infected people—such a compound is referred to as a *lead compound*. Not surprisingly, the high costs associated with developing a new antiviral drug are reflected in the final cost of the drug to the user.

Once laboratory experiments have developed a potential antiviral compound to the point where it shows promise as an anti-HIV drug, clinical trials in humans are conducted. Clinical trials are typically conducted in the following sequence:

Phase I clinical trials are conducted on a small number of individuals, and they simply determine the safety of the compound (toxicity or side effects) and establish the methods needed to deliver useful concentrations of the drug into the body. *Phase I trials do not test for effectiveness of the compound.* They are often conducted on uninfected individuals.

Phase II clinical trials are limited in size and test whether the compound has effectiveness (efficacy). In the case of trials for antiviral drugs, efficacy might be measured by a reduction in symptoms (see Table 6–5), a reduction in laboratory measures of viral infection, or an increase in measures of immune function (see below). Phase II trials are conducted in HIV-infected individuals.

Phase III clinical trials are large-scale efficacy trials of the compound. They are typically conducted in multiple locations, and the efficacy of the compound is compared to the efficacy of the currently available therapies. Compounds must show efficacy in Phase III clinical trials before they can receive approval by the Food and Drug Administration (FDA) for prescription as an antiviral drug. Prior to that time, the compounds are considered *experimental* drugs.

Biomedical researchers devote a great deal of effort to developing new antiviral drugs, but it is also important to improve existing drugs. In particular, improvements in the existing formulations of the drugs are beneficial. As described in Chapter 5, p. 108, taking the current antiviral therapies for HIV is very complicated, particularly for individuals taking the combination therapies. Adhering to the strict routines of the combination therapies becomes a major part of the daily existence of HIV-infected individuals. If improved formulations of the antiviral drugs are developed (for instance, development of time-release capsules that decrease the number times a drug must be taken), they will improve the quality of life.

As described in Chapter 5, the development of the protease inhibitors and their inclusion in combination therapies in 1996 sparked a great deal of optimism. Since, in some individuals, the combination therapies have reduced the viral RNA loads in the blood below the levels of detection, some scientists have proposed that it might be possible to completely eradicate HIV infection from an infected individual. If this were to occur, then the individual could stop taking antiviral drugs. However, this should be viewed only as a hope at this time. In particular, while the combination therapies rapidly eliminate viral RNA from the blood, virus persists for considerably longer in the lymph nodes. HIV-infected macrophages probably persist much longer than HIV-infected T_{helper} lymphocytes, because they are not killed by the virus (see Chapter 4, p. 64). In addition, HIV can establish latent infections that might reactivate years later.

Another potential class of antivirals is the set that interferes with the ability of the virus to enter cells. If the virus entry process is inhibited, then spread of infection within an individual might be inhibited. As discussed in Chapter 4, HIV virus particles initially attach to cells by way of the cellular receptor CD4 protein that is imbedded in the surface of normal T-lymphocytes and macrophages. Recombinant DNA techniques have been used to make large amounts of a part of pure CD4 protein. Test-tube experiments showed that if this CD4 protein fragment is incubated with T-lymphocytes or macrophages and HIV, the CD4 protein fragment could bind to the HIV before it binds to the cells. Thus, it could prevent HIV infection of the cells. However, when versions of this CD4 protein fragment were tested in clinical trials, they did not prevent further infection in HIV-infected individuals.

As also discussed in Chapter 4, cells require a co-receptor in addition to CD4 protein for binding and infection by HIV. Therefore, scientists have recently focused on blocking the co-receptor interaction with HIV as a way of preventing infection. There is reason to believe that this approach may be effective. A small percentage of the human population completely lacks the CCR5 co-receptor (involved in infection of macrophages) because of a naturally occurring genetic mutation. Epidemiological studies have found that these individuals are quite resistant to HIV infection after repeated exposures through sexual contact. Thus, an antiviral drug targeted at the CCR5 co-receptor may also be effective in preventing spread of HIV infection. The first generation of co-receptor blocking compounds is nearing clinical trials.

As time passes, new potential antivirals will continually appear—some from pharmaceutical laboratories and some from nontraditional sources. They initially spark great interest, typically based on anecdotal reports of effectiveness. It is important to subject these compounds to rigorous scientific testing (clinical trials; see above) to determine if they work as claimed. If not, they could worsen the conditions of HIV and AIDS patients who abandon traditional and proven therapies in favor of the new compounds. In the past, one compound that attracted considerable interest was GLQ223, or Compound Q. This drug is derived from a Chinese herbal medicine (from bitter cucumber), and it was found to kill HIV-infected cells in culture. However, standard clinical trials have not definitively proven GLQ223's effectiveness. In addition, serious neurological side effects, including coma, have occurred in some individuals taking GLQ223 in early clinical trials. Thus, interest in this compound has declined.

Two new classes of potential antiviral agents have recently been developed out of basic molecular biology research. One class of compounds is called *antisense* molecules. These are small pieces of single-stranded DNA or RNA that can specifically form double-stranded complexes with HIV viral RNA, similar in structure to double-stranded DNA. Formation of these double-stranded complexes can lead to destruction of the viral RNA. As a result, an infected cell cannot produce viral RNA, viral protein, or virus particles. Current research is focused on establishing methods to effectively deliver these antisense molecules to infected cells and determining which antisense molecules (directed against which regions of the viral RNA) are most effective.

The other class of potential antiviral compounds is called *ribozymes*. Ribozymes are very specialized antisense RNA molecules. When they combine with HIV RNA, they attack the HIV RNA and cut the strand at particular sites. Thus, they can inactivate virus expression.

Restoration of the Immune System

Most of the clinical symptoms in AIDS result from failure of the immune system, due to depletion of T_{helper} lymphocytes. If the immunological defects can be repaired, then the disease might be arrested or even reversed. As discussed in Chapter 3, all cells of the blood (including those of the immune system) arise by division and differentiation from stem cells that are located in the bone marrow. This process is controlled by a complex series of growth factors that circulate in the body, as described in Chapter 3. Blood cell growth factors are currently the subject of a great deal of research—they are important in many other diseases in addition to AIDS. Ultimately, it may be possible to use these growth factors to stimulate and regenerate the immune system in AIDS patients. Of course, it will be important to use these growth factors in conjunction with antivirals. Otherwise, continued HIV infection would destroy the immune system again. Another potential complication is that growth factors may directly or indirectly activate HIV from latently infected cells.

One growth factor that has shown promise in restoring the immune system in HIV-infected individuals is IL-2 (interleukin 2) (see Chapter 3, p. 46). This is logical, since IL-2 is required for growth of both T_{helper} and T_{killer} lymphocytes. A clinical trial on HIV-infected individuals with low T_{helper} lymphocyte counts showed substantial increases in T_{helper} cells after a series of intravenous IL-2 infusions. During this trial, the patients were also treated with antiviral compounds to prevent spread of any latent HIV that was reactivated by the IL-2. However, there are two major drawbacks to this potential treatment. First, IL-2 is an extremely powerful biological molecule. When administered intravenously it can cause severe side effects, including very high fevers and shock. Patients often receive IL-2 treatment in a hospital setting in order to manage the side effects. Second, IL-2 therapy will be very expensive: the IL-2 itself is very expensive, and hospitalization costs add to the overall cost of the therapy. It would be difficult to provide the current IL-2 therapy to large numbers of HIV-infected people. However, the positive results obtained with IL-2 provide encouragement for developing other, more economical and manageable ways to stimulate the immune systems of HIV-infected individuals.

In addition to naturally occurring growth factors for the immune system, several artificial substances that may be able to stimulate immune system regeneration are being developed and tested.

Another possible approach to restoring the immune system would be to supply an AIDS patient with functional T-lymphocytes. Technically, this is very difficult to accomplish because mature T-lymphocytes do not divide. Instead, as described in Chapter 3, it would be necessary to provide new blood stem cells that can divide and differentiate into functional T-lymphocytes. The most logical way to supply these stem cells is through a bone marrow transplant, in which uninfected bone marrow cells are implanted into the recipient individual. These bone marrow cells could then produce functional T-lymphocytes. The greatest technical problem with this approach is that HIV in the infected individual can infect the transplanted bone marrow and destroy the resulting T-lymphocytes. Current cutting-edge research is focused on developing ways to make bone marrow cells resistant to HIV before transplanting them—for instance, by implanting them with an anti-HIV ribozyme (see above).

Treatment of Opportunistic Infections and Cancers

The major practical problems for AIDS patients generally are the opportunistic infections (OIs) and cancers that result from the lack of immunological protection. Thus, development of better therapies for these OIs and cancers will play an important role in improved treatment of AIDS patients.

In terms of opportunistic infections, it will be necessary to develop effective drugs for each different OI. Many of these infections were rather rare before the AIDS epidemic, since the causative agents generally do not cause disease in healthy individuals. As a result, little effort had been put into developing drugs for them. For example, at present, no effective treatment can control cryptosporidiosis as an opportunistic infection. The only recourse right now is to treat the symptom (diarrhea). Continued efforts need to focus on developing drugs for these OIs.

In addition to new drugs, improved methods of delivery are also being developed. As an example, pentamidine is one of two treatments used for pneumocystis pneumonia. Intravenous treatment with pentamidine is the standard procedure, but many patients experience side effects from the drug. Researchers have found that inhalation of a pentamidine mist brings the drug directly to the lungs and is very effective in treating PCP. At the same time, the side effects of the drug are reduced because it is delivered only to the area of infection (the lungs) and not to other regions of the body that may experience side effects. Aerosol pentamidine is also used preventively in HIV-infected individuals who have low T_{helper} lymphocyte counts, but who have not yet developed PCP.

The cancers that result from HIV infection range from Kaposi's sarcoma to tumors of the immune system, called *lymphomas*. These cancers are quite distinct diseases, and different therapies will be necessary for each of them. In the case of Kaposi's sarcoma, one treatment involves use of a naturally occurring protein called alpha-interferon. Cancer researchers may also provide new therapies for the cancers associated with AIDS. A compound that has recently been used for treatment of Kaposi's sarcoma is taxol. Taxol was first used in the treatment of ovarian cancer.

Modifying the Conduct of Clinical Trials

Treating HIV-infected individuals often involves new or experimental drug therapies. The AIDS crisis has led to some modifications in the typical clinical trial procedures used for licensing drugs in the United States. The FDA oversees drug licensing, and it requires extensive testing in laboratory animals and humans before a drug is approved for therapy. This is a very time-consuming and expensive process, typically taking many years. Largely due to pressure from AIDS activist groups, several modifications in these procedures have been developed to speed drug testing and also to make experimental drugs available to patients during the approval process. Traditionally, experimental drugs are administered only through official clinical trials, which usually take place in university research hospitals. To expand the availability of these trials to more patients, *community-based trials* have been established in which experimental drugs are administered to AIDS patients by their local physicians. These physicians then report the results of the treatment to a central source, where the results are pooled.

Another problem with standard clinical trials is that some individuals are too far away from a research university to participate in a trial. As a result, *parallel track* procedures have been developed, in which an experimental drug is made available to a patient (through his or her doctor) in parallel with a clinical trial if that patient is unable to obtain access to the drug otherwise.

Another way AIDS clinical trials have been modified is through the development of *surrogate endpoints*. In clinical trials, the standard yardsticks (endpoints) used to judge a drug's effectiveness are development of clinical disease or death. However, this presents a problem for HIV and AIDS, since the time course of infection and disease is so long. When disease or death are used as the endpoints, a clinical trial of an AIDS drug could take many years. As a result, other measurements of an individual's immune system or health have been substituted in preliminary evaluations of HIV drugs. The most common surrogate endpoints are a patient's CD4 (T_{helper}) lymphocyte count, the amount of viral protein (p24 antigen) detectable in the blood, and the viral RNA load in the blood. If a drug lowers the amount of circulating viral RNA or protein or if it increases the T_{helper} lymphocyte count, it would be provisionally considered effective. In fact, the decisions to approve DDI, DDC, and the protease inhibitors as anti-HIV drugs were partly based on clinical trials with surrogate endpoints. However, the accuracy of different surrogate endpoints in reflecting the overall clinical state of HIV-infected individuals is still open to debate.

FUTURE DIRECTIONS FOR SOCIAL EFFORTS

Infectious diseases do not affect only isolated people. On the individual level, the spread of an infectious agent is caused by the interactions of individuals within a society. On the community level, everyone is directly or indirectly living with AIDS. Therefore, in combating infectious diseases, it is important to consider society as a whole in planning solutions. This is particularly important for diseases such as AIDS, for which there is currently no cure or vaccine. Social efforts related to AIDS can make contributions in two main areas: education and research.

Education

The two aspects of education that can have significant effects on different parts of the AIDS epidemic are education for prevention and education for understanding and compassion.

Education for Prevention

Educational programs targeted to members of high-risk groups are extremely important. These programs are the key to making these individuals aware of the dangers they face and also to promoting changes in behavior that will lessen the risks. As described in Chapter 2, the experience with the syphilis epidemic earlier this century shows the effectiveness of proper public health measures. As also discussed in Chapter 2, public health measures effectively limited the last plague outbreak at the turn of this century—even at a time when there was no cure for the disease. This is analogous to our present situation with AIDS. However, changing individual attitudes and behaviors is a challenging task.

In the context of AIDS, public health education has been strongly endorsed by the National AIDS Commission. As discussed in Chapter 7, safer sex recommendations have been developed to reduce the risk of spreading HIV infection through sexual relations. It will be very important to develop effective programs of education and behavior modification to persuade high-risk individuals to adopt safer sex practices. Addressing HIV infection in injection drug users is an extremely critical issue, because these individuals may be the conduit for spread of infection into the general heterosexual population. The current programs have had limited success and they are underfunded.

Development and implementation of public health measures targeted to injection drug users will be challenging. For instance, as mentioned in Chapter 7, there are pilot programs to distribute clean needles to drug addicts, in order to reduce the risk that users will share a contaminated needle with someone else. Such programs have been opposed by some people who argue that distribution of needles condones and encourages drug addiction.

Development of public health programs to combat AIDS will also require particular attention to ethnic groups. As described in Chapter 6, African Americans and Hispanics represent a disproportionate number of AIDS patients. This is particularly true for HIV-infected individuals who are injection drug users— more than 75 percent of AIDS patients who acquired the disease through injection drug use are African American or Hispanic. Public health programs targeted to these groups will be very important.

Another important goal of public health education will be to prevent backsliding in behavior. Behavior modification through public education has clearly been effective in areas where the AIDS epidemic has hit hard—for instance, the gay male community in San Francisco. However, recent follow-up studies have detected a significant frequency of reversion to high-risk sex practices by some men in this community as time has passed. It will be important to develop methods to promote continued adherence to safer behaviors, even after initial efforts have been effective.

Education for Understanding and Compassion

Another aspect of education is equally important: educating the general public about HIV, AIDS, and those with the disease. Fear and lack of knowledge and experience have fostered prejudice and discrimination against those with HIV and AIDS. Education of various types and in various forms can help to lessen the fear of HIV and AIDS by increasing knowledge about what HIV is, how it is spread, and how it is medically treated. In addition, as knowledge grows, it will be easier to develop and implement public policies to decrease discrimination against those with HIV and AIDS and to increase programs to stop the spread of the disease.

Health care workers are another important target for educational efforts. The number of doctors who treat HIV-positive individuals and people with AIDS (PWAs) has grown, but it still remains small in comparison with the need. Additional educational programs are necessary to address concerns of doctors and other health care workers. Some special clinics or wards in hospitals have made treating PWAs their specialty. In these cases, the quality and sensitivity of care for people living with AIDS has been much better than that generally available. The lessons learned from these settings need to be disseminated to other health care workers so that more HIV-positive individuals and PWAs can benefit.

From the discussion in Chapter 6, we know that more and more individuals will either be infected with HIV or progress from HIV-positive status to AIDS status. The increases in numbers of individuals affected by the disease will strain our current health care and social service systems. For the wisest decisions to be made about the allocation of scarce financial and personnel resources, we need to have a general population that is informed about HIV and AIDS. The decisions will be difficult enough without fear and prejudice clouding the public's consideration of options.

Research

All of these education efforts rely on good research. Whether we are developing HIV prevention programs for individuals or AIDS education programs for the general public, we need to draw on the research and theories available to us. For example, the development of effective HIV prevention programs requires careful and detailed attention to a number of factors, such as cultural and social aspects of people's situations. Good social research will allow us to identify these factors and determine which approaches will most likely be effective.

We also need to improve our epidemiological and survey research related to AIDS. As AIDS has moved into new communities, our epidemiological research has been slow to catch up. For example, AIDS has begun to appear in the Asian/Pacific Islander community in the United States. Initially, epidemiological data grouped these individuals in the "other" category, instead of the more frequently chosen racial and ethnic categories (Anglo, Hispanic, African American, etc.) Now, Asian/Pacific Islander is listed separately under racial and ethnic groups. As the AIDS epidemic has continued to spread in this community, however, a more detailed breakdown is needed. The cultural practices and beliefs are different enough between Asian/Pacific Islander subgroups that, for effective prevention planning, we need to know more about exactly which subgroups are most affected by HIV.

Likewise, we need accurate survey research on HIV- and AIDS-related knowledge, attitudes, and practices among different segments of the population. We have thorough survey research on certain special study groups of PWAs (for instance, gay men), which has been invaluable in planning and implementing both biomedical and psychosocial programs. Our research on other segments of the population affected by HIV is less complete or missing. For example, we have limited research on injection drug users and their HIV attitudes and practices, and we have very little or almost no systematic research on certain subgroups (such as sex workers) and HIV. Without good research, we are unable to develop a thorough understanding of the HIV-related context and the individuals and factors within it.

Finally, we need better evaluation of all of our HIV and AIDS programs. Only through scientific research can we be sure that we are implementing programs with beneficial effects. Too often, we establish a program with the best of intentions but without a sound scientific plan to assess the actual effects or to detect unintended consequences, both positive and negative. Scientific evaluation provides those working to address the social aspects of AIDS with a way to know if their efforts are effective. Decreases in HIV infection rates are the ultimate outcome of many prevention programs. Unfortunately, we cannot always measure this outcome, and even if we could, HIV infection rates change slowly over a long period of time. For the most complete picture, we need to assess changes in knowledge, attitudes, intentions, practices, and HIV status.

A FINAL NOTE OF OPTIMISM: TIME IS ON OUR SIDE

Many of the facts and statistics about AIDS in this book are frightening and depressing, especially since a cure has not been developed yet. Indeed, those who are suffering from the disease or at risk to develop it often express frustration at the apparent lack of progress in AIDS research. But let's look at some time scales to get a sense of perspective. First, as discussed in Chapters 4 and 6, the current estimates are that most HIV-infected individuals will develop AIDS with an average time between initial infection and disease symptoms of eight to ten years, even if they do not receive antiviral drugs. Thus, new therapies and treatments that are developed in the next five or ten years may be able to help many of those who are currently infected.

Second, let's look at the rate of scientific progress in the AIDS epidemic. For comparison, let's consider two other diseases that have had great impacts on society: the ancient disease, plague (black death), and the more recent disease, polio (see Chapter 2). Table 8–1 compares the time scales for fighting these diseases.

Table 8–1
A TIME COMPARISON OF THREE EPIDEMICS

Disease	First Documented Epidemic	Isolation of Agent	First Therapy
Plague (*Yersinia pestis*)	A.D. 560	1894	1940s (antibiotics)
Polio (poliovirus)	A.D. 1885	1909 identified 1949 isolated	1953 (Salk vaccine)
AIDS (HIV)	A.D. 1981	1984	1986 (AZT partially effective)

Plague probably first caused major epidemics as early as the fifth or sixth century A.D.; the well-documented black deaths occurred in the fourteenth and following centuries A.D. The infectious agent, *Yersinia pestis,* was finally isolated in 1894. Effective therapy against the disease had to wait for the development of classical antibiotics in the 1940s.

Polio was first recognized as an epidemic disease in the 1880s, and the infectious agent, poliovirus, was isolated in the late 1940s. Even after the virus was identified, there was no effective therapy for individuals once they became infected. Ultimately, the disease was brought under control by the development of the Salk and Sabin polio vaccines beginning in 1955.

As for AIDS, the disease was first recognized in 1981 and the causative agent, HIV, was isolated in 1983–1984. By the end of 1986, the first partially effective antiviral, AZT, was developed; it was put into wide use in 1987. The protease inhibitors and triple combination therapies were introduced in 1996, and they provide a significant improvement in the management of HIV-infected individuals. Indeed, the introduction of the triple combination therapies, or HAART, in 1996 has led to a decrease in the rate of death from AIDS in those countries that have access to these drugs. For instance, as shown in Table 8–2, in the United States there was a 45 percent decrease in deaths from AIDS in the first

Table 8–2
AIDS CASES AND DEATHS IN THE USA: 1996 VS. 1997[1]

	January–June 1996	January–June 1997	% Decrease 1997–1996
Total AIDS Cases	33,243	28,370	15%
Total AIDS Deaths	21,281	11,479	45%

[1]Data taken from the CDC. Protease inhibitors and the triple combination (HAART) therapies were introduced in mid-1996, so January–June 1996 represents the last period before introduction of these therapies.

half of 1997 as compared to the first half of 1996 (the triple combinations became available in mid-1996). Similarly, as shown in Figure 8–1, the number of the new AIDS diagnoses in Canada markedly declined between 1995 and 1997. (In this case, it is important to remember that this does not mean that the number of HIV-infected people has decreased or that the rate of new HIV infections has decreased; the decline is related to the ability of the triple combination therapies to inhibit progression of HIV-infected people to AIDS.) Unfortunately, recent reports indicate that the decrease in AIDS deaths in 1998 was only about half the decrease observed in 1997 (see Chapter 5). Thus, the rate of progress in AIDS research has actually been very rapid in historical terms.

The progress in AIDS biomedical research largely reflects the great advances in molecular biology, virology, immunology, and biotechnology that have taken place over the last 25 years. For instance, the life cycle of retroviruses was worked out largely in the 1970s, after the discovery of reverse transcriptase. In terms of immunology, the understanding of the different kinds of lymphocytes (B versus T; T_{killer} versus T_{helper}) is also quite recent. The techniques to identify the CD4 protein of T_{helper} lymphocytes are less than 15 years old. It is difficult to imagine how much more serious the AIDS epidemic would be if it had struck 30 years ago, before these advances. One program that provided a major boost to these fields was the War on Cancer, which was a program launched by the U.S. government to conquer cancer with the same approach used to put a man on the moon. While the War on Cancer has not been won yet, the program resulted in a great deal of

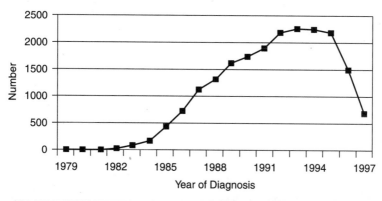

Figure 8–1

The yearly number of AIDS diagnoses in Canada is shown. This graph is taken from a report, *The Status and Trends of the HIV/AIDS Epidemic in the World,* issued by UNAIDS in June 1998.

research on retroviruses, and it heavily contributed to the development of recombinant DNA cloning technologies. This has been essential to the rapid achievements in AIDS research. Because biomedical research has advanced so rapidly in the last few years we are optimistic that new and more effective solutions to HIV and AIDS will be developed in the not-too-distant future.

In personal terms, there are positive approaches we all can take to dealing with the AIDS epidemic. Because death is an inevitable part of the lives of all of us, it is more productive to focus on wellness and the quality of life than on illness and death. This applies both to those who have AIDS and those who do not—as well as to people affected by cancer or other terminal illnesses. Like all major social changes, AIDS presents us with not only problems but also opportunities on both biomedical and social levels. For example, we have already expanded our scientific knowledge of the immune system due to the efforts to understand AIDS. We also have a better understanding of the important factors in successful disease prevention and health promotion programs. There are many other opportunities to make progress on biological and social issues. AIDS is a crisis and an opportunity for social improvement: The challenge is to use the opportunities for greater personal, social, and biological understanding.

GLOSSARY

AIDS Acquired immune deficiency syndrome is an incurable infectious viral disease that results in damage to the immune system in otherwise healthy individuals.

AIDS antibody test A test to determine whether an individual has antibodies to HIV, the virus that causes AIDS. Presence of HIV-specific antibodies indicates that the person has been exposed to HIV and has raised an immune response, but it does not tell if the person is still infected. The most common test is the ELISA test. A backup test called the Western blot is also used.

Analytical epidemiology Epidemiological studies that seek to identify and explain the causes of diseases.

Anemia A condition of the blood in which there are abnormally low concentrations of red or white blood cells.

Antibiotics Compounds that are effective against infection by microorganisms such as bacteria, fungi, and protozoa. They are generally ineffective against virus infections.

Antibody A protein produced by a B-lymphocyte that specifically binds a particular antigen. This leads to attack by the immune system.

Antigen A molecule or substance against which a specific immune response is raised.

Antisense molecules DNA or RNA molecules that can form specific double-stranded couples with HIV RNA. They can bind to HIV RNA and prevent it from functioning in the infected cells and are being explored as therapeutics for HIV infection.

Antivirals Compounds that are effective in treating virus infections.

Asymptomatic AIDS carriers Individuals infected with HIV who do not show any sign of disease. They may be capable of infecting others.

Asymptomatic infection An infection for which there are no superficially visible or noticeable changes in the body or its functions that would indicate the presence of the infection. (Contrast with **Symptomatic disease.**)

Azidothymidine (AZT) Also called retrovir or zidovudine. An antiviral that is effective in treating HIV infection and AIDS. It works by preferentially being incorporated by reverse transcriptase into growing viral DNA during HIV replication.

Bacteria Small single-cell microorganisms that can cause diseases.

B-lymphocytes One kind of lymphocyte. B-lymphocytes secrete antibodies that are specific for particular antigens.

Case/control studies A form of analytical epidemiology in which a group of individuals with a particular disease (the cases) are compared to a matched group of unaffected individuals (the controls).

Case reports Reports and descriptions of an unusual disease occurrence in individual patients. Case reports are one form of descriptive epidemiology.

Causality The factors contributing to the development of disease in epidemiological studies.

CD4 protein A surface protein that is characteristic of T_{helper} lymphocytes. It is also present on some macrophages and dendritic cells. CD4 protein is the cell receptor for HIV.

Cellular immunity Immunity involving T-lymphocytes (particularly T_{killer} lymphocytes).

Circulatory system The system of vessels that moves blood around the body, including arteries, veins, and capillaries.

Clades Subgroups of HIV. Various human populations throughout the world are infected by different clades of HIV. In North America, the predominant subgroup of HIV-1 is clade B.

Clinical trial Trials of drugs, vaccines, or therapies in humans. They are the final tests used before the treatments are approved for public use.

Cohort studies A form of analytical epidemiology in which a group of individuals who share a particular risk factor for a disease are studied.

Control group A group of individuals who serve as the scientific comparison for a similar but separate experimental group of individuals who receive a special treatment or intervention. The presence, meaning, and significance of changes in the experimental group due to the special treatment or intervention are identifiable through comparisons with the control group. See also **Experimental group.**

Co-receptors for HIV Cell surface molecules required along with surface CD4 protein for HIV binding and infection of a cell. The two predominant HIV co-receptors are CCR5 and CXCR4. CCR5 is the co-receptor found on macrophages, and CXCR4 is the co-receptor on T_{helper} lymphocytes.

Combination therapies (also triple combination therapies or AIDS drug cocktails or HAART) Combinations of antivirals administered to HIV-infected individuals. They have been found to be considerably more effective than single antiviral drugs alone in giving sustained reductions in viral RNA load. Also called *HAART.*

Cross-sectional/prevalence studies Monitoring a population for occurrence of diseases and noting the time and kind of disease. A form of descriptive epidemiology.

Dementia Loss of mental function due to damaged brain cells and brain inflammation in AIDS-afflicted patients.

Descriptive epidemiology Epidemiological studies that describe the occurrence of disease by person, place, and time. Generally the first kinds of studies carried out in a new disease.

Drug-resistant HIV Virus that frequently appears in HIV-infected individuals taking an antiviral drug. Once a drug-resistant HIV appears, then that antiviral drug is no longer effective in that person.

ELISA The most common test for HIV antibodies.

Endemic pattern Patterns of continuous infection that allow epidemic diseases to remain present in populations.

Epidemiology The study of patterns of disease occurrence in populations and the factors affecting them.

Experimental group A group of individuals who receive a special treatment or intervention and who are compared with a control group of similar but separate individuals. See also **Control group.**

Experimental/interventional studies A form of analytical epidemiology in which a condition in a population is changed, and the effect on disease development is observed.

Fungi Microorganisms that may exist as single cells or be organized into simple multicellular organisms.

Germ theory The postulate (1546) that infectious bacterial, fungal, or viral organisms cause disease.

HAART Highly active antiretroviral therapy. A combination of antiretroviral drugs that efficiently inhibit HIV replication in infected individuals. Typically the combinations include two nucleoside inhibitors and one protease inhibitor. These are also called triple combination therapies or AIDS drug cocktails.

Helper T-lymphocytes T-lymphocytes that help T_{killer} and B-lymphocytes respond to antigens. Destruction of T_{helper} lymphocytes is the major problem in AIDS.

HIV (Human Immunodeficiency Virus) The virus that causes AIDS; previously called HTLV-III, LAV, and ARV. The predominant form of HIV in North America, Europe, and central Africa is HIV-1. A closely related retrovirus found in western Africa is HIV-2.

Humoral immunity Immunity involving B-lymphocytes and the antibodies they produce.

IDU Injection drug user.

Immune system The circulating cells and serum fluids in the blood that provide continuous protection from foreign infectious agents.

Immunological memory The ability of the immune system to respond rapidly to a previously encountered antigen with specific antibodies.

Incidence The proportion of a population that develops new cases of a disease during a particular time period.

Incubation period The period between infection by a microorganism and appearance of disease symptoms.

Interleukin 2 (IL-2) A growth factor required by T lymphocytes. It is produced by stimulated T_{helper} lymphocytes and is required by both T_{helper} and T_{killer} lymphocytes for growth.

Kaposi's sarcoma A normally rare cancer that develops frequently in AIDS patients.

Killer or cytotoxic T-lymphocytes T-lymphocytes that kill the target cells they bind to.

Koch's postulates A series of criteria used to establish that a particular microorganism causes a disease.

Latency A state of virus infection in which the virus's genetic material remains hidden in the cell, but no virus is produced. At a later time, the latent virus may become reactivated. HIV can establish latent infection, particularly in macrophages.

Lead compound A compound in drug development that shows activity against HIV in a laboratory culture. It may be modified by a pharmaceutical chemist to make even more effective antiviral compounds, some of which may eventually be useful in management of HIV infection in people.

Lentiviruses A subclass of retroviruses that includes HIV. Some lentiviruses infect other species, including monkeys, sheep, and cats.

Lymphadenopathy syndrome (LAS) Persistently enlarged lymph nodes or swollen glands, sometimes an early sign of HIV infection that is progressing. Also called PGL (persistent generalized lymphadenopathy).

Lymphatic circulation A second circulatory system that lymphocytes circulate through. Lymph channels drain fluid from tissues (lymph) into lymph nodes, where B- and T-lymphocytes are located. Antibodies or T-lymphocytes are produced in the lymph nodes in response to infection, and they enter the general circulation by way of other lymph channels.

Lymphocytes Cells of the immune system that respond specifically to foreign substances. There are several kinds of lymphocytes. The two classes of lymphocytes are B-lymphocytes and T-lymphocytes.

Lymphoma Cancer of lymphocytes of the immune system.

Lytic infection Infection of a cell by a virus that results in death of the cell. HIV infection of T_{helper} lymphocytes is a lytic process.

Macrophages One kind of phagocyte. Macrophages generally attack cells infected with viruses.

Nonlytic infection Infection of a cell by a virus that results in production of virus, but survival of the cell. Most retroviruses normally carry out nonlytic infections. HIV infection of macrophages is nonlytic.

Non-nucleoside Reverse Transcriptase Inhibitors (NRTIs) Anti-HIV drugs targeted to the HIV reverse transcriptase but distinct from the nucleoside analogs. NRTIs bind directly to the viral reverse transcriptase and directly inhibit its action.

Nucleoside analogs A class of antiviral drugs that inhibit HIV replication. They are incorporated by reverse transcriptase into the growing viral DNA molecule, but once incorporated they prevent further growth of the viral DNA. AZT was the first nucleoside analog approved for treatment of HIV-infected people. Five nucleoside analogs have been approved for treatment in HIV/AIDS: AZT, DDC, DDI, D4T, and 3TC.

Opportunistic infections Infections by common microorganisms that usually do not cause problems in healthy individuals. OIs are the major health problems for AIDS patients.

Pandemic disease An infectious disease present on many continents simultaneously.

Phagocytes Cells of the immune system that eat foreign cells or infected cells. The two kinds of phagocytes are macrophages and neutrophils (granulocytes).

Phase I clinical trials The first clinical trials carried out during development of a drug or a treatment. Phase I clinical trials test for toxicity, and they establish the methods for achieving effective doses of the drug or treatment. They do not test for effectiveness (efficacy).

Phase II clinical trials Limited clinical trials that test for efficacy of the drug or treatment.

Phase III clinical trials Large-scale clinical trials that test for efficacy in multiple settings and compare the efficacy of a drug or treatment with the currently available drugs/treatments.

Polymerase chain reaction (PCR) A sensitive method for detecting the presence of a specific DNA or RNA. PCR-based assays have been developed for detection of HIV viral DNA and RNA. They are the basis for the HIV viral RNA load assays.

Prevalence The fraction of individuals in a population who have a disease or infection at a particular time.

Primary immune response The immune response that follows first-time exposure to an infection or an antigen. There is a lag period before antibodies are produced.

Protease An enzyme encoded by HIV and other retroviruses. It is important in maturation of the virus particle and is required for infectivity.

Protease inhibitors Antiviral drugs that inhibit HIV protease. They have become important drugs for management of HIV infection, particularly when used in triple combination therapies with nucleoside analogs.

Protozoa Large single-cell microorganisms that can cause diseases.

PWA Person with AIDS.

Quarantine Enforced isolation of individuals with an infectious disease or of individuals suspected of having an infectious disease.

Red blood cells (erythrocytes) Blood cells that are responsible for carrying oxygen and carbon dioxide to and from the tissues.

Reverse transcriptase An enzyme that is unique to all retroviruses. It reads the genetic information of the retrovirus, which is RNA, and makes a DNA copy.

Ribozymes Specialized forms of antisense RNA molecules. They can cause the cutting of HIV RNA in infected cells and are being explored as potential therapeutic molecules for HIV infection.

Secondary immune response An immune response that follows exposure to an infection or an antigen that the immune system had encountered before. The strength of the subsequent response is greater, occurs more rapidly, and lasts longer.

Seronegative An individual who tests negative for HIV antibodies.

Seropositive An individual who tests positive for HIV antibodies.

SHIV Hybrid simian-human immunodeficiency virus. SHIVs are generated in the laboratory and consist of an HIV gene substituted into SIV for the equivalent SIV gene. Useful SHIVs are those that replicate and/or cause disease in primates.

Simian immunodeficiency virus (SIV) A group of retroviruses closely related to HIV that are native to old world (African) primates. Some SIVs cause AIDS when infected into particular primates species. SIVs are often used as experimental models for HIV. HIV-1 is most closely related to SIV from chimpanzees, and HIV-2 is most closely related to SIV from sooty mangabeys.

Surrogate endpoint Indicators of the effectiveness of drug therapies that substitute for the standard indicators (i.e., development of disease or death). For HIV, surrogate endpoints are measures of the condition of an individual's immune system such as CD4 lymphocyte counts, the amount of viral protein (p24 antigen) in the blood, and viral DNA load.

Susceptibility Capacity of a person to be infected by or to be unresistant to a disease.

Symptomatic disease A disease for which there are superficially visible or noticeable changes in the body or its functions that indicate the presence of the disease. These changes are unpleasant or harmful and thus call attention to the consequences of the disease. (Contrast with **Asymptomatic infection**.)

Test group See **Experimental group**.

T-lymphocytes One kind of lymphocyte. Unlike B-lymphocytes, T-lymphocytes do not release antibodies, but they specifically recognize and bind foreign antigens. There are two main types of T-lymphocytes: T_{killer} and T_{helper} lymphocytes.

Treatment adherence The ability of a person taking a therapy to follow the prescribed treatments. Treatment adherence is a serious concern in triple combination therapies of HIV-infected people.

Vaccine A preparation that can induce protective immunity to a microorganism such as a virus or bacterium. Some vaccines are inactivated or attenuated microorganisms, and others consist of purified proteins of the microbe.

Viral envelopes Structures that surround some virus particles and resemble membranes around cells. Viral envelopes contain virus-specific proteins that are important in binding cell receptors. Viral envelope proteins are major targets for the immune system.

Viral RNA load (or **viral load**) The amount of HIV RNA detectable in the blood of an infected person. This reflects the amount of HIV virus particles in the blood. Viral RNA load measurements employ the PCR reaction, which is very sensitive. They are much more sensitive for detecting HIV infection than either ELISA assays for HIV antibodies or assays for viral p24 antigen.

Viruses Small infectious agents. They are parasites that must grow inside cells.

Western blot An HIV antibody test, used as a confirmatory test for a positive ELISA test.

White blood cells (leukocytes) All blood cells except red blood cells, including lymphocytes, neutrophils, eosinophils, macrophages, and megakaryocytes.

Window period For an individual, the period of time between infection by a virus and the production of antibodies to the virus.

Xenophobia Discriminatory fear of foreigners.

APPENDIX

REFERENCE RESOURCES

HIV/AIDS is a continually evolving topic. New biomedical and social developments happen almost daily. This appendix provides the reader additional sources to find the latest information on HIV/AIDS.

Web Sites

A great number of HIV/AIDS Web sites can provide the latest scientific, medical, and social updates. If a Web site does not have the information desired, checking linked Web sites is recommended. Several well-organized and maintained Web sites are:

CDC Division of HIV/AIDS Prevention:
http://www.cdc.gov/nchstp/hiv_aids/dhap.htm
U.S. Centers for Disease Control Web site—has latest epidemiological statistics; downloadable slides on HIV/AIDS.

CDC National Prevention Information network:
http://www.cdcnpin.org/
CDC Web site focused on prevention of HIV infection.

UNAIDS: http://www.unaids.org/old/
United Nations AIDS program Web site. Excellent for the global AIDS perspective.

HIV/AIDS Treatment Information Service:
http://www.hivatis. org/
and
HIV/AIDS Clinical Treatment Information Service:
http:www. hivactis.org/
Two linked Web sites that provide up-to-date information on HIV/AIDS treatments and clinical trials.

AIDS Education Global Information System (AEGIS):
http://www.aegis.com/
An extremely comprehensive AIDS Web site, covering all aspects of AIDS; updated hourly.

New York Times: http://www.nytimes.com/
Searchable Web site for the *New York Times.*

Los Angeles Times: http://www.latimes.com/
Searchable Web site for the *Los Angeles Times.*

Johns Hopkins AIDS Service: http://www.hopkins-aids.edu/
An excellent university-based Web site.

AIDS Science and Society/Biology of AIDS Web site:
http://www.jbpub.com/AIDS
A Web site established by Jones & Bartlett Publishers to support
this book.

AIDS Information and Discussion:
http://4aids.com
A commercial Web site with HIV/AIDS information notable for
its discussion group chat rooms.

Books

Abbas, A. K., A. H. Lichtman, and J. S. Pober. (1997). *Cellular
and Molecular Immunology.* Philadephia, PA: W. B. Saunders.
An advanced/graduate-level text in immunology.

Benjamini, E., G. Sunshine, and S. Leskowitz. (1996). *Immunology—A Short Course,* 3rd ed. New York: Wiley-Liss.
A college-level immunology text.

Coffin, J. M., S. H. Hughes, and H. E. Varmus, eds. (1997).
Retroviruses. Plainview, NY: Cold Spring Harbor Laboratory
Press.
The authoritative graduate/professional-level reference book on
retroviruses. It includes extensive discussion of HIV.

Stine, Gerald. (1998). *Acquired Immune Deficiency Syndrome,*
3rd ed. Upper Saddle River, NJ: Prentice-Hall.
An entry-level college text on HIV/AIDS; contains many facts.

INDEX

The abbreviations *t* and *f* stand for table and figure, respectively.